Medicare Meltdown

OTHER BOOKS BY ROSEMARY GIBSON
AND JANARDAN PRASAD SINGH

Wall of Silence
The Treatment Trap
The Battle Over Health Care

Medicare Meltdown

How Wall Street and Washington Are Ruining Medicare and How to Fix It

Rosemary Gibson and
Janardan Prasad Singh

ROWMAN & LITTLEFIELD PUBLISHERS, INC.
Lanham • Boulder • New York • Toronto • Plymouth, UK

Published by Rowman & Littlefield Publishers, Inc.
A wholly owned subsidiary of The Rowman & Littlefield Publishing Group, Inc.
4501 Forbes Boulevard, Suite 200, Lanham, Maryland 20706
www.rowman.com

10 Thornbury Road, Plymouth PL6 7PP, United Kingdom

British Library Cataloguing in Publication Information Available

Library of Congress Cataloging-in-Publication Data

Gibson, Rosemary, 1956–
Medicare meltdown : how Wall Street and Washington are ruining Medicare
and how to fix it / Rosemary Gibson and Janardan Prasad Singh.
   pages cm
Includes bibliographical references and index.
  ISBN 978-1-4422-1979-3 (cloth : alk. paper) — ISBN 978-1-4422-1980-9
(electronic)
   1. Medicare—Finance. 2. Medicare—Forecasting. 3. Health care reform—
United States. I. Singh, Janardan Prasad, 1960– II. Title.
  RA412.3.G53 2013
  362.1068'1—dc23   2012042960

♾️™ The paper used in this publication meets the minimum requirements of
American National Standard for Information Sciences—Permanence of Paper
for Printed Library Materials, ANSI/NISO Z39.48-1992.

Printed in the United States of America

To the one who inspires every moment every day.

Contents

Acknowledgments

This book would not have been possible without our many friends and colleagues in American medicine and nursing who have helped us understand the changes taking place on the front lines of twenty-first-century health care. They have shown us where the ground is shifting beneath our feet.

We are especially grateful for the wisdom of friends in the Consumers Union Safe Patient Project who have shared their individual and collective wisdom as patients and advocates for improvement in the quality and safety of the nation's health care. They have peeled back the veneer and traced the impact of the business of American medicine on the decisions made, the products used, how long a doctor or nurse spends with a patient, and most assuredly, the cost of it all. We weave together the wisdom of many to reveal a big picture that is right in front of us, invisible, yet ever so powerful in shaping Medicare's future and health care for us all.

We are indebted to those who blew the whistle to tell the inside story about the influence of Wall Street on Medicare policy making in Washington. What they know and shared with us is never written in any Washington health-policy newsletters or textbooks. They are courageous people, quintessential public servants who challenged the status quo when it was incompatible with the interests of seniors and other Americans. They bear the scars of being truth tellers in a world where the powerbrokers spare no effort to quash the truth and the people who tell it.

Our purpose is to give voice to those who have no voice, who lie awake at night worried about being sick, wondering what to do. Our aim is public policy that serves the public interest, not any special interest.

If this book accomplishes nothing else, we hope that it reveals a different path to protect and sustain a program that is a veritable lifeline for millions of people. The path we point to is not the easiest way forward and perhaps the hardest. But it is the right way.

We are deeply indebted to Dr. Larry Jassie for his unerring enthusiasm and for reading multiple drafts. Sarveshwari Singh and Shriansh Singh provided invaluable research assistance on fast-changing events surrounding Medicare.

We have no words to express our heartfelt appreciation to Suzanne Staszak-Silva at Rowman & Littlefield, who understood the importance and timeliness of the book and what it means for seniors, boomers, and the country's future. We are truly honored and delighted to work with her to bring it to fruition.

Introduction

$\mathcal{W}$e write this introduction in the first year of President Barack Obama's second term in the White House, as the clock ticks on the automatic spending cuts and tax increases, otherwise known as the "fiscal cliff." Once again, Washington is a battleground over how to get the nation's fiscal house in order.

Looming in the background is Medicare, the cherished program that protects Americans from the infirmities of old age and the financial ravages of American-style health care. The prospect of increasing the Medicare eligibility age from sixty-five to sixty-seven raises its unwelcome head. Meanwhile, optimal policy proposals to remove the waste that litters the program are buried deep in Washington's political backyard.

We bring out of the shadows options to protect Medicare that would have overwhelming public support. You, the reader, have a right to know there are ways to protect Medicare without shifting an overwhelming burden to the public.

This book brings a new vantage point to the debate over how to protect Medicare for today's seniors, boomers, Gen X, Gen Y, and beyond. It shines a light on the rarely seen side of the program—the business of Medicare.

Most people think of Medicare as an entitlement for older Americans. Medicare is also big business. Hospitals, drug companies, device manufacturers, and other enterprises rely on Medicare for nearly six hundred billion dollars in annual revenue, which is the amount that the program spends in a year.

Today, fifteen health care companies are on the Fortune 100 list. When Medicare was enacted in 1965, there were none. A new health care industry was inaugurated when President Lyndon Johnson signed Medicare into law. It grew with vigor and stamped its own expansive footprint on the nation's economy and politics.

The health care enterprise has brought life-saving products and services to Americans. But the metamorphosis of Medicare into a program whose biggest clients include corporate giants has turned the storied program on its head. They have an outsized impact on the care that seniors, boomers, and all Americans receive, and they are a powerful force shaping the future of the program.

In part I, we introduce Medicare with fifteen surprising facts about this popular federal program. It explains where the money comes from to pay for Medicare, who pays, and how much. A clear message is that many boomers need to be prepared to pay a substantial—and growing—share of their future income for health care. As Democrats and Republicans spar over Medicare's future, we compare and contrast their ideas to sustain Medicare and what they mean for seniors' pocketbooks. More fiction than fact swirled during the 2012 presidential campaign, and we sort the facts from the fiction.

In part II, we go behind the scenes to show where the nearly six hundred billion dollars that Medicare spends in a year actually goes, who gets it, and how they are looking to get more of it. It begins with the real-life story of a Kentucky man who received a bill for one night in the hospital that cost as much as a house in his community. We explain the forces driving up the cost of a hospital bill. The story is emblematic of Medicare's biggest challenge. We crack open the myth that health care in America costs so much because it is the best in the world. Lay readers and savvy policy makers will learn something new about Medicare and where it is headed.

In part III, we take a close look at the business of Medicare. The program's abundance has attracted newcomers from private equity firms and hedge funds. They are buying hospitals, hospices, and other health care facilities, and their business practices have permanently altered Medicare's culture and the care that seniors receive. The political landscape in Washington has changed too, with these new players on the scene who will be a powerful force in crafting Medicare's future. Recent tangles surrounding Medicare that have played out behind the scenes on

Capitol Hill provide a preview for what seniors and boomers can expect. Meanwhile, what happens on Wall Street doesn't stay on Wall Street. It trickles down into day-to-day experience, affecting life in ways as basic as getting out of bed in the morning.

Republicans are avid proponents of curbing what they call the culture of dependence on government that people have become accustomed to. Both parties are silent, however, about the culture of dependence on Medicare that health care businesses have become accustomed to.

As a lucrative program for some of the biggest companies in the world, Medicare revenue permeates the balance sheets of firms big and small. They depend on constantly growing revenue from Medicare to meet unforgiving demands from their owners for bigger, better, quicker returns. This culture of dependence has infused many nonprofit hospitals and other health care facilities.

The culture of dependence on Medicare among U.S. businesses has created an entitlement mindset. It is on a direct collision course with the need to reduce the federal government's debt, a course that threatens the country's financial solvency.

The Institute of Medicine of the National Academy of Sciences reports that 30 percent of Medicare spending is wasted on unnecessary medical care, inefficient delivery of care, fraud, and abuse. A solution to sustain Medicare is to tighten the spigot on the wasteful spending that flows to businesses that make money from it.

Does Washington have the gumption to do it? In part IV, we name the seven habits of the highly entitled health care industry. As with any entitlement, there are givers and takers, the entitlers and the entitled, the elected officials and the health care industry. The ties are strong between Washington policy makers and Wall Street investors. We shine a light on how they advance each other's interests. We reveal how most of the candidates during the 2012 presidential campaign had a track record of strengthening the industry's access to more of Medicare's money.

Medicare's future will be a tug-of-war. It won't be between guns and butter—that is, between military spending and Medicare. As skirmishes in Washington have already demonstrated, it will be between a health care industry that is programmed to take more for itself and the people this storied program is meant to serve. This is the epic battle that will be waged for Medicare's future, and with it the health and well-being of seniors and every American who is counting on it.

Democrats say that Republicans will end Medicare as Americans have known it. The truth is that the strong ties forged by both Democrats and Republicans that bind Wall Street and Washington have already put Medicare on a path to meltdown. The course can be changed, but it requires action—fast.

The purpose of this book is to open up the debate and reveal a different path that can be taken to ensure Medicare's future. President Obama and Republicans have proposed raising Medicare's eligibility age from sixty-five to sixty-seven, saving about fifteen billion dollars a year while shifting an enormous and unacceptable burden to older Americans.

If the president and Republicans cut a mere 15 percent of the more than one hundred billion dollars that Medicare wastes annually on improper payments (forty-eight billion dollars) and fraud (sixty billion dollars), equivalent savings could be generated. Commonsense solutions such as this are rarely presented because business interests narrow the options for Medicare's future to serve their own advantage.

In part V, we conclude with a vision to restore Medicare to its original purpose, which is to serve the people who work hard to pay for it and who hope that Medicare will be there for them. By shoring up Medicare, Americans from all walks of life will be healthier and wealthier, and America will be too.

Democracy can never be taken for granted. It confers a duty upon citizens to be informed. Knowledge guided by wisdom must precede action. That is why we wrote this book. Each and every generation must learn and practice it anew to balance the excesses of the political and business elite. Otherwise, it will be lost, and once it is gone, the road to reclaim it is long and arduous, and more often than not, unsuccessful.

Medicare will celebrate its fiftieth birthday in 2015. When the history books are written fifty years from now, we want historians to say that once upon a time, Americans from all walks of life had access to some of the best medical care in the world because of Medicare. Its creators were generous beyond measure. As Medicare reached middle age and everyone took stock of its past, present, and future, they realized that a midcourse correction was needed. Changes were made and Medicare remained intact, keeping the promise to the people whose beloved program, and the security it confers, lives on.

Our aim is to offer a way to achieve this vision. We wrote this book for boomers, seniors, and everyone else who pays for Medicare from their weekly paychecks and Social Security income. You are Medicare's rightful owners and have a right to know the actors who are shaping Medicare's future and their script. You can participate in the country's democracy armed with information about what the fight for Medicare's future is really all about.

For policy makers in the federal government, we hope this book will give you a fresh and compelling perspective on how Medicare can be protected for older Americans and everyone else who pays for it.

We hope this book will help citizens and policy makers in other countries who are grappling with ways to create a financially sustainable health care system. For leaders in emerging markets such as India, Brazil, and China where health care spending is growing exponentially, we hope you can learn from the good aspects of Medicare's design and implementation and avoid its pitfalls.

The measure of a country's wealth is the health of its people. In the end, that is the measure by which Medicare should be judged. It is not how much money it makes for Fortune 100 companies or Wall Street investors, or how many votes it can win in an election. Only then can Medicare serve its noble purpose.

Rosemary Gibson
Janardan Prasad Singh
Winter 2013

Part I

HOW MUCH IS MEDICARE COSTING YOU?

Follow the money. That's what we do in this first part of the book. Chapter 1 gives a brief flyover of the Medicare program with fifteen fascinating facts about how much you pay for Medicare and the value of the benefits you can expect to receive. We dispel myths about where the money comes from to pay for Medicare and reveal where the U.S. government borrows money to pay today's Medicare bills. We shine a light on surprising features of the program that you won't read anywhere else.

For seniors on fixed incomes, money matters. Chapter 2 reveals the astonishing increase in how much seniors spend from their Social Security checks to pay for Medicare. The outlook for boomers who have yet to retire is more of the same. An ever-increasing amount of boomers' Social Security income will be spent on Medicare, leaving less money to spend on housing, food, and other necessities of life. Meanwhile, many seniors continue to grapple with aftershocks from the stock market collapse that triggered the Great Recession in 2008, when twelve trillion dollars in market value was lost, wiping out hard-earned retirement savings.

Chapter 3 gives a candid picture of why the status quo in Medicare cannot continue. The numbers tell the story. Its spending trajectory is, literally, off the charts. This interpretation is not a Democratic or Republican perspective. We dissect the proposals of each political party to strengthen Medicare's finances and explain what they mean for seniors. They differ in fundamental ways. Nonetheless, similarities exist because there are only so many ways that Medicare can be on a path of financial sustainability. We take a look at how the health care reform law, the Patient Protection and Affordable Care Act, affects Medicare.

In chapter 4 we predict the impact of Medicare's fiscal challenges on the care seniors and boomers will receive in coming decades. Seniors will be caught in the middle of a demographic bulge and inevitable curbs on growth in Medicare spending. The impact is already evident. Newly eligible boomers are learning that not all doctors accept Medicare, and if they want to stay with their favorite doctor, they may need to pay the cost themselves. In the name of efficiency, health care is becoming a commodity. Patients are widgets. Time to talk with a doctor or nurse is being engineered out of visits to the doctor and hospital stays. Seniors and boomers who are looking ahead to retirement are in for a big squeeze. So are doctors and nurses who will care for them.

Fifteen Medicare Facts
That Will Astonish You

If you are reading this book, Medicare is probably a part of your life. If you have turned sixty-five, you depend on it. If you are a young boomer, you are counting on it to protect you when you retire. If you are part of Gen X or Gen Y, you contribute to Medicare from your paycheck. Whether rich or poor, young or old, or somewhere in between, nearly everyone is touched by Medicare.

If you have good genes and are a boomer, you might be wondering whether Medicare will be around in twenty-five years. If you are just starting out in your career, you are probably wondering whether you can count on Medicare when you reach age sixty-five.

Here are fifteen Medicare facts that will surprise you. They give a preview of where Medicare is headed and what it means for you.

FACT #1: IF MEDICARE WERE A COUNTRY, IT WOULD BE THE TWENTIETH LARGEST ECONOMY IN THE WORLD.

Medicare is a huge program, and it spent $560 billion in 2011. This amount is larger than the entire economy of Sweden and more than double the size of Ireland's economy.

FACT #2: MEDICARE WASTES THE EQUIVALENT OF THE ENTIRE ECONOMY OF NEW ZEALAND.

The Institute of Medicine of the National Academy of Sciences reported that 30 percent of the money spent on health care in the United States does not add value to the health of Americans. It is wasted on overtreatment, inefficiencies, and poor management. For Medicare, this means that about $170 billion doesn't help seniors. This amount is more than the entire economy of New Zealand, whose gross domestic product—the value of all the goods and services it produced that same year—was $162 billion.

FACT #3: BETWEEN NOW AND 2030, MEDICARE WILL BE ADDING THE EQUIVALENT OF THE POPULATIONS OF AUSTRIA, HONG KONG, ISRAEL, AND SWITZERLAND TO ITS ROLLS.

Today, about forty-nine million people are covered by Medicare. By 2030, thirty-three million more people will be on Medicare. This is equivalent to adding more than the entire current populations of Austria, Hong Kong, Israel, and Switzerland.

FACT #4: TEN THOUSAND BOOMERS SIGN UP FOR MEDICARE EVERY DAY.

Medicare is facing a giant demographic wave. Ten thousand baby boomers will turn sixty-five every day for the next twenty years and be eligible for Medicare. This is an important reason, but not the only one, that Medicare's financial future is on shaky ground.

FACT #5: THE AVERAGE PERSON PAYS SIXTY THOUSAND DOLLARS FOR MEDICARE DURING A LIFETIME OF WORK.

Sixty thousand dollars is a lot of money. It will pay for in-state tuition for four years of college at the University of Michigan or a year at Harvard. Many Americans will work more than a year to earn that amount. It is also the amount of money deducted for the Medicare payroll tax from the average American's paycheck during a lifetime of work.

FACT #6: A NEW RETIREE CAN EXPECT TO RECEIVE ABOUT $180,000 IN MEDICARE BENEFITS.

Medicare is a good deal for seniors. Consider Steve, a sixty-five-year-old printer who earned about $43,500 a year during his working life. When he retired in 2011 at age sixty-five, his lifelong contribution to Medicare from payroll taxes totaled about $60,000, and he can expect to receive nearly three times that amount, or about $170,000 worth of medical-care benefits, according to estimates by the Urban Institute, a Washington, DC, think tank. His twin sister, Susan, earned about the same amount and worked the same number of years, and she will receive about $188,000 in medical benefits because as a woman she will likely live longer than her brother and use more medical care.

Congressman Jim Cooper from Tennessee introduced a bill in Congress to require Medicare to send an annual statement to each person with his or her total payroll tax contributions and an estimated value of expected benefits. Congress did not act on this commonsense idea.

FACT #7: YOUR FEDERAL INCOME TAXES PAY FOR A GROWING SHARE OF MEDICARE'S COSTS.

If a senior receives about $180,000 in benefits but pays only $60,000 in payroll taxes, where does the rest of the money come from to close the gap? There are myths and facts about where the money comes from. But first, here are the ABCs of Medicare.

Think of Medicare as a birthday cake with multiple layers. The first layer, Part A, pays for overnight hospital care, skilled nursing home care, and hospice.

The second layer, Part B, pays for physician, hospital outpatient, home health care, and other services.

Part C is a private plan option called Medicare Advantage that seniors can choose instead of traditional Medicare. These plans are offered by companies such as Kaiser Permanente and UnitedHealthcare. Part C combines both Part A and Part B. Part D provides subsidized coverage for outpatient prescription drugs.

When economist Paul Krugman wrote a column in the *New York Times* about Medicare, a reader responded with the following comment:

> In my opinion, federal programs such as Social Security and Medicare that are supported by participants' insurance premiums and not by federal general tax revenues should not be a political football in Congress. While these programs need to be reviewed for their future sustainability, they have not contributed to the current federal debt.

The reader who wrote the comment was not correct. Here is where the money comes from to pay for benefits that seniors receive.

Medicare payroll tax revenue collected from workers covers only about 38 percent of Medicare's total costs. The tax is 2.9 percent of income and the money is used to pay for Part A hospital and other care.

When seniors are on Medicare, they pay premiums for hospital outpatient care and doctor visits (Part B) and prescription drugs (Part D). The premiums cover about 13 percent of Medicare's total costs.

Most remaining costs, 44 percent, are paid by federal income taxes. So workers pay for Medicare twice every payday. They pay the Medicare payroll tax and federal income tax. In fact, Medicare is becoming more reliant on incomes taxes to pay its bills.

Medicare contributes to the federal debt because the federal government doesn't collect sufficient money from income taxes and other sources to pay all its bills. It borrows the remaining money and pays interest on the debt that accumulates. So, yes, Medicare contributes to the federal government's debt.

FACT #8: THE NUMBER OF CORPORATE HEALTH CARE FIRMS ON THE FORTUNE 100 LIST HAS INCREASED FROM ZERO IN 1965 TO FIFTEEN TODAY.

Since the Medicare program was established in 1965, health care has become a big business. The number of for-profit health insurers, hospitals, hospices, imaging centers, ambulatory surgery centers, and companies that make and sell medical devices, drugs, and hospital supplies has grown dramatically. Not all of them make it to the Fortune 100 list, but here are the big-league companies: McKesson, CVS Caremark, Cardinal Health, UnitedHealth Group, Walgreens, Medco, Pfizer, Johnson & Johnson, WellPoint, Merck, Express Scripts, Abbott Laboratories, Humana, Aetna, and HCA.

Here is another indicator of health care as big business. Seventy-six percent of Fortune 50 companies have a connection to the health care industry and increasingly rely on Medicare and other insurers for a share of their revenue and profits.

FACT #9: BEFORE YOU CALL YOUR STOCK BROKER, READ THIS: THE FEDERAL GOVERNMENT BORROWS MONEY FROM CHINA TO PAY MEDICARE BILLS FROM HOSPITALS, DOCTORS, AND DRUG COMPANIES.

People who invest in the stock market might be excited to know that the health care industry will be booming in the coming years. A growing share of money will come from an unusual source. The federal government does not have the cash on hand to pay all the $1.6 billion a day in bills that Medicare receives from hospitals, doctors, hospices, home-care agencies, and all other providers. The federal treasury borrows money from China and other lenders to pay many of its bills, including Medicare, adding to the government's debt. For now, the U.S. Treasury can borrow money at low interest rates. When money is cheap, spending borrowed money is easier. Sooner or later, the cost to borrow money will become expensive.

FACT #10: PRESIDENT OBAMA AND RUSH LIMBAUGH AGREE ON THIS FACT.

President Obama and conservative radio talk show host Rush Limbaugh agree on one thing about Medicare. President Obama said, "The U.S. government is not going to be able to afford Medicare . . . on its current trajectory. . . . The notion that somehow we can just keep on doing what we're doing and that's OK, that's just not true." Meanwhile, Limbaugh said, "I don't like the idea of letting Medicare collapse. I think it's already happening." When political polar opposites agree on something, it must be true.

FACT #11: THE HEALTH CARE INDUSTRY WILL REAP
FROM MEDICARE A LARGER SHARE OF THE COUNTRY'S
GROSS DOMESTIC PRODUCT BETWEEN NOW AND 2035.

For the foreseeable future, Medicare will be taking a larger bite from
the country's income from all the goods and services it produces—its
gross domestic product, or GDP. The companies that rely on Medicare
for their revenue will be taking a larger share of the country's income,
too. This means that the federal government will have less money to
pay for other essentials that a country needs to function: infrastructure,
investments in science and technology, education, and national security,
among other priorities.

FACT #12: THE NUMBER OF DOCTORS WHO
SPECIALIZE IN CARING FOR SENIORS IS
SHRINKING WHEN MORE ARE NEEDED.

As the number of baby boomers on Medicare soars, the number of doctors who specialize in caring for older people in the field of geriatrics
is shrinking. They help keep seniors healthy, out of the hospital, and
on as few drugs as possible. In 2010, only seventy-five young doctors
who graduated from medical school in the United States and went into
internal medicine and family medicine chose to do additional training in
geriatrics, a decline from 112 in 2005. The median salary of geriatricians
is lower than that of almost all specialties even though they provide an
immensely valuable service to the nation's seniors. Ironically, Medicare
is the primary source of taxpayer money for training doctors. One of the
greatest threats to the health and well-being of America's burgeoning senior population is the lack of doctors and other health care professionals
who specialize in the care of older adults.

FACT #13: MEDICARE'S MONEY FOR
HOSPITAL CARE BEGINS TO RUN OUT IN 2024.

Beginning in 2024, the money to pay for hospital care under Medicare
Part A won't be enough to cover expenses, according to Medicare

trustees who issue a nonpartisan, just-the-facts annual report on the program's finances. Medicare will have only enough money to pay 90 percent of the expected cost of hospital care for seniors.

Here is what the Medicare trustees wrote, "If assets were exhausted Medicare could pay health plans and providers only to the extent allowed by ongoing tax revenues—and these revenues would be inadequate to fully cover costs. Beneficiary access to health care services would rapidly be curtailed." Congress has never allowed hospital funds to become depleted. But where will the money come from to close the gap?

The federal government has issued official warnings since 2007 about Medicare's pending financial insolvency as required by the Medicare Modernization Act of 2003. The first warning was issued by Michael O. Leavitt, Secretary of Health and Human Services under President George W. Bush, who wrote, "The Medicare program is on an unsustainable path, driven by two principal factors: projected growth in its per-capita costs and increases in the beneficiary population as a result of population aging."

More warnings have been issued since then. In 2012 Secretary of the Treasury Timothy Geithner and other trustees warned of "disruptive consequences" if action is not taken to stem Medicare's red ink.

FACT #14: 79,200 MEDICARE BENEFICIARIES DIE EACH YEAR BECAUSE OF PREVENTABLE HARM IN HOSPITALS.

When doctors were asked by the U.S. Department of Health and Human Services to review the medical records of seniors to determine the quality of care they received, they found that many seniors are harmed by preventable mistakes and other causes. They estimate that 79,200 Medicare beneficiaries a year die because of harm in hospitals that could have been prevented.

FACT #15: ANNUAL MEDICARE FRAUD AND ABUSE IS EQUIVALENT TO THE LIFETIME MEDICARE CONTRIBUTIONS FROM ONE MILLION SENIORS.

The Federal Bureau of Investigation estimates that up to 10 percent of the money Medicare spends each year, or nearly sixty billion dollars, is lost to fraud. This amount is equivalent to taking the sixty-thousand-dollar lifetime Medicare contributions from about one million middle-income seniors every year and giving it to criminals. Medicare officials and prosecutors in the U.S. Department of Justice are eager to stop it, but the sheer scale of fraud is so extensive that it exceeds the authority and resources that Congress appropriates to combat it.

That's not all. Another category of misuse of Medicare money is called "improper payments." They occur when mistakes are made in coding payments and calculating the amount of money Medicare owes. Improper payments also include those made to doctors and hospitals for surgeries or other treatments that are medically inappropriate and can cause more harm than good. They are not considered fraud because evidence of intent to defraud Medicare can be difficult to prove. Medicare estimates that it made forty-eight billion dollars in improper payments in 2010.

In the pages that follow, we tell you more about where your money goes, who is getting it, what they are doing with it, and how Medicare can be put on a more financially sustainable path without cutting benefits or raising the Medicare eligibility age.

They're Coming for
Your Social Security

Comedian and social commentator the late George Carlin said to a New York audience, "They're coming for your Social Security money. . . . You know, they'll get it. They'll get it all sooner or later."

Carlin was referring to Wall Street firms that wanted Social Security to be privatized so they could earn fees from managing the money. President George W. Bush proposed to partially privatize Social Security. During the 2000 presidential campaign, he described how it would work, saying, "A young worker can take some portion of his or her [Social Security] payroll tax and put it in a fund that invests in stocks and bonds."

Bush initially proposed privatization after the stock market had a good run in the 1990s. In 1995 the Dow Jones Industrial Average topped five thousand points. Less than four years later, in an unprecedented run-up in stock prices, the Dow jumped a whopping six thousand points to reach more than eleven thousand points in May 1999.

Banks and investment firms were eager to manage even a small share of Social Security money. Every month Social Security benefits worth about fifty billion dollars are sent to America's retirees. Firms that manage employee 401(k) pension plans charge anywhere from 6 percent of the amount of money in employee accounts to less than 0.1 percent. If banks and financial investment firms could garner even 0.1 percent of the fifty billion dollars in Social Security benefits paid each month, they would make fifty million dollars a month, or more than half a billion dollars a year.

Bush's opponent, Al Gore, the former vice president and senator from Tennessee, raised red flags about privatizing Social Security. During a presidential debate in 2000, Gore said, "Your future [Social Security] benefits would be cut by the amount that's diverted into the stock market. And if you make bad investments, that's too bad."

After the 2000 election, Bush continued to advocate for privatizing Social Security. In an interview on CNBC in 2006, he said, "A worker at his or her option ought to be allowed to put some of their own money into a private savings account, an account they can call their own. They'll get a much better rate of return on their money than they would in Social Security if the government managed it. . . . This is asset accumulation which is good for American families."

The luster of the stock market had worn off by then, blackened by the 40 percent drop in the Dow during the dot-com bust in 2002 and 2003. By October 2006, the Dow had crawled back to twelve thousand points.

In the run-up to the 2008 presidential election, the market tanked and trillions of dollars in retirement savings were wiped out. On March 9, 2009, the Dow dipped below 6,500 points, losing nearly half of its value from its peak.

If Bush had been successful in partially privatizing Social Security, younger workers who had opted to divert a portion of their Social Security payroll taxes into stocks would have joined the millions of Americans who lost a large share of their retirement savings. In fact, they would have taken a double hit. Their contributions and any market gains would have been decimated. Financial services firms would have been the only ones to make money from fees to manage the accounts.

The stock market has regained ground lost during the Great Recession, but individual investors are at an enormous disadvantage. High-frequency traders dominate the market now, using powerful computers and complex algorithms to comb the market in search of quick profits. Wild swings in the Dow Jones Industrial Average scare away average individual investors, who realize they don't stand a chance of winning, any more than a pedestrian walking along a NASCAR race course would still be standing at the end of a race.

Enterprising minds continue to look for ways to claim a larger share of retirees' Social Security checks. Here is how they are doing it. If you work, you are like most Americans and receive the white-and-green Social Security statement every year that estimates how much you can expect to receive in Social Security benefits when you retire.

The average Social Security benefit for a retired person is $1,175 per month. If you are counting on receiving all of it each month to use for groceries and living expenses, you need to read this. If you sign up for Medicare when you reach age sixty-five, the cost of the premium for insurance to cover hospital outpatient care and doctor visits (Part B) is deducted from your Social Security check. You will not see that money.

In 2000 the premium was only about fifty dollars a month, or 5 percent of the average Social Security check. By 2010, premiums more than doubled to $110.50, which is equivalent to about 9 percent of the average Social Security check. Seniors with higher incomes paid more. That's not all. If you went to the doctor, you paid an annual deductible of $155 and a 20 percent copayment for each visit.

If you sign up for Medicare Part D to cover the cost of prescription drugs, you will pay a monthly premium of about thirty dollars for a standard private prescription drug plan. You may pay a copayment for drug purchases too. Your premium will cover only about 25 percent of the cost of the drugs. The federal government uses federal income tax revenue to pay the remaining cost.

When all the out-of-pocket costs for Part B and Part D are added, 27 percent of the average Social Security check in 2010 was used to pay for doctor visits and prescription drugs, according to the Medicare trustees who oversee the program, as shown in figure 2.1. This amount applies to people who had average incomes when they worked. If you

Figure 2.1.   Percent of the Average Social Security Check Needed to Pay for Medicare Part B and Part D Premiums and Co-Pays

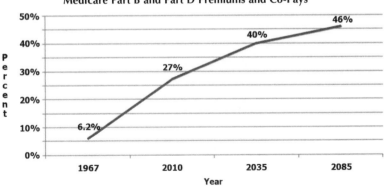

Source: Medicare Trustees Report

have a very low income, you will receive help to defray the cost. Most seniors who have traditional Medicare pay for supplemental insurance, called Medigap, that covers many of the cost-sharing requirements.

As boomers sign up for Medicare, health care will take an even larger bite in years to come. In twenty years, when the first boomers reach age eighty-five, the cost of Part B and Part D will consume more than one-third, or 36 percent, of the Social Security checks of people who had a modest income during their working years.

If a newly retired boomer lives to the ripe old age of ninety, he or she will pay more than 40 percent of his or her Social Security for premiums and copayments for doctor visits and prescription drugs. By the year 2085, their cost will consume nearly 50 percent of the average Social Security check.

Social Security is the largest source of income for many people over age sixty-five, so the financial burden of health care will increase if nothing is done to change course. Supplemental health insurance coverage to defray the out-of-pocket costs will become more expensive too.

Health care is taking a larger share of Social Security checks because the prices for a hospital stay, brand-name drugs, and everything else have been increasing so steeply. The number of doctor visits, tests, surgeries, and drugs that people are being prescribed is going up too. When price and volume increase simultaneously, a double whammy drives up spending.

In Medicare's early days, a senior paid only 6.2 percent of Social Security income for Medicare Part B. There was no Part D prescription drug coverage at that time.

If you are admitted to the hospital, you will pay an additional amount. Hospital insurance (Part A) has no premium if you are eligible for Social Security, but you will pay an annual deductible and copayments. In 2011 the annual deductible was $1,132. A copayment of 20 percent of the cost for each day is required too. About one in five people on Medicare are hospitalized each year and are affected.

George Carlin's prediction was right. Social Security income is being whittled away. Hospitals, health insurance companies, drug and device firms, and all others who rely on Medicare for their revenue and profit are going to the bank with a larger share of seniors' Social Security income.

Will Democrats and Republicans Really Fix Medicare for You?

$\mathscr{I}$f you have been paying for health care, you know that premiums and out-of-pocket costs are taking a larger slice of your income. Meanwhile, Medicare is taking an ever-increasing share of the country's income.

If Medicare spending continues to grow at the same pace relative to the growth in the country's income, by 2082 Medicare will consume nearly 25 percent of the value of all the goods and services the nation produces, according to the Congressional Budget Office, as shown in figure 3.1. Seniors and boomers can't afford to spend 25 percent of their income on Medicare. Neither can the country.

If health care spending for everyone in the United States is included, not just Medicare, and if it keeps growing at the same pace

Figure 3.1. Projected Medicare Spending as a % of GDP Based on Historical Spending

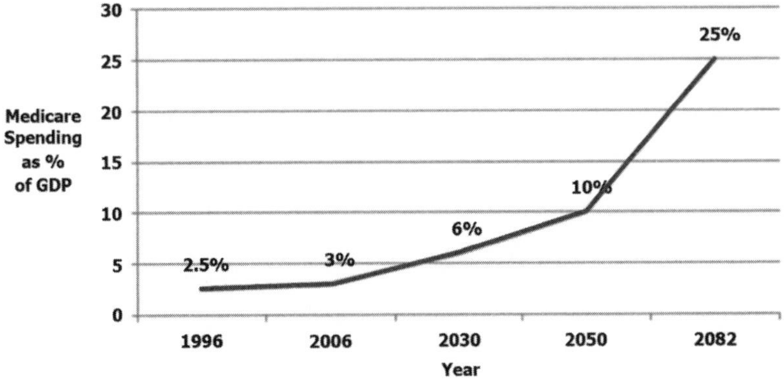

Source: Congressional Budget Office

Figure 3.2. Projected Total Health Care Spending as a % of GDP Based on Historical Spending

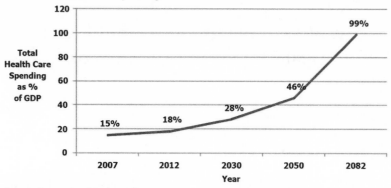

Source: Congressional Budget Office

relative to the country's income, health care will consume virtually all the nation's income, 99 percent, by 2082, as shown in figure 3.2. This projection is tucked away in an appendix of a 2007 report by the Congressional Budget Office.

All long-term spending projections are riddled with the possibility of errors in assumptions about events that will take place seventy years from now. Nonetheless, projections of future spending based on actual historical spending relative to income reveal that business as usual is untenable.

Policy makers will not allow health care spending to crowd out all other spending on infrastructure, defense, homeland security, and other vital public goods. That is why official projections from the federal government for Medicare spending are much lower. They assume that government will act to bend the cost curve. Still, official projections may be too optimistic. The 2012 Medicare trustees report stated, "Actual future Medicare expenditures are likely to exceed the intermediate projections, possibly by quite large amounts."

HOW HEALTH CARE REFORM AFFECTS MEDICARE

During the 2012 presidential campaign, Mitt Romney claimed that Barack Obama's health care reform will "gut" Medicare. Obama claimed that the Republican plan will "end Medicare as we've known it." Who is right? First, let's take a look at how health care reform, the Patient Protection and Affordable Care Act, changed Medicare.

New Medicare Benefits for Seniors

The reform law added benefits to Medicare as a way to garner support from seniors. Medicare now pays for mammograms and colonoscopies with no copayment, and seniors can have a free annual wellness visit to their doctor.

The gap in prescription drug coverage, or the "donut hole," will be closed by 2020. The gap has required seniors to pay the full cost of their prescriptions out of pocket if their spending levels reached certain thresholds. Seniors didn't need to wait long after President Obama signed the health care reform law to receive a tangible benefit. Shortly afterward, nearly four million beneficiaries received a $250 check to defray their costs when they reached the donut hole. Seniors also receive a 50 percent discount on brand-name drugs when they reach the coverage gap.

More Money to Reduce Medicare Fraud

The health care reform law added $350 million over ten years to ramp up the fight against Medicare fraud. The fraud fighters have new authority to prevent fraud rather than "pay and chase," which has been the norm. Still, the added investment is minuscule in relation to the nearly sixty billion dollars in fraud that is drained from Medicare every year. Also, the law cannot create the political will to prosecute fraud perpetrated by special interests.

Higher-Income Earners Pay Higher Medicare Taxes and Premiums

The Medicare payroll tax is 2.9 percent on all wages, with employers and employees each paying 1.45 percent. Under the law, high-income individuals are paying another 0.9 percent on earned income over $200,000, or $250,000 if married.

High-income earners are paying a new 3.8 percent tax on net investment income, including interest, dividends, and capital gains.

Also, higher-income seniors are paying higher premiums for Medicare Part B for hospital outpatient services and doctor visits. Together, these three provisions are expected to raise $318 billion in revenue from 2013 to 2022.

Hospitals and Other Providers Receive Lower Annual Payment Increases

Hospitals and other health care providers will continue to be paid more under Medicare, but their annual increases will be less. The change is similar to an employee who gets a salary increase every year but the amount of the raise will be less than expected. The total reduction in payments to health care providers is $415 billion over ten years, according to the Congressional Budget Office. Hospital cuts will be $260 billion; skilled nursing facilities, $39 billion; hospice services, $17 billion; home health services, $66 billion; and for all other providers, $33 billion.

The conservative *Washington Examiner* mused that hospitals will stop participating in the program. This is unlikely because hospitals receive about 30 percent of their revenue from Medicare, so they are not going to abandon it. Many will increase the volume of procedures and tests performed on seniors to make up for the reduction in payment.

Hospitals will shift more of their costs to employers and employees with private insurance. This response is not mere speculation. The Maryland Hospital Association proposed to state regulators in 2012 that private health insurers that operate in the state pay more to hospitals to offset Medicare payment cuts and cuts in the state's Medicaid program. Residents of Maryland who have private coverage could pay an extra nine hundred dollars per hospital admission based on initial estimates.

Under the reform law, Medicare Advantage plans are receiving lower payments. Medicare has been paying more money for a senior who was enrolled in a private plan compared to the amount it would have paid if the senior had been in traditional Medicare. Total reductions will be $156 billion over ten years.

MEDICARE AND THE 2012 PRESIDENTIAL CAMPAIGN

With Mitt Romney's selection of Paul Ryan, a Republican congressman from Wisconsin, as his running mate, Medicare took center stage in the 2012 presidential campaign. It resurrected criticisms of Ryan and fellow Republicans who proposed in 2011 to dramatically restructure Medicare.

Paul Ryan said in 2011 before the presidential campaign revved up that traditional Medicare should end. In his original proposal, he wanted all future retirees under age fifty-five to choose a private insurance plan. Traditional Medicare would be phased out. Seniors would be given a set amount of money every year, called a defined contribution, to choose a private health plan, which is a fundamental change from traditional Medicare, which pays directly for all the services that doctors, hospitals, and others provide.

Ryan was blunter than most elected officials about Medicare's dire straits. "If you wait and allow the political paralysis to stop us from fixing and saving this program . . . then you're going to have severe disruptions in seniors' lives that would just be, I think, morally wrong because we see this problem coming," he said. Democrats criticized Ryan's original plan because it would end Medicare as it is today. This assessment is accurate. Medicare would be fully privatized in about thirty years and cease to exist as the country has known it.

Within the Republican party, Newt Gingrich publicly excoriated Ryan's original plan on *Meet the Press*, saying,

> I don't think right-wing social engineering is any more desirable than left-wing social engineering. I don't think imposing radical change from the right or the left is a very good way for a free society to operate. I think we need a national conversation to get to a better Medicare system with more choices for seniors. . . . I think that this is too big a jump. I think what you want to have is a system where people voluntarily migrate to better outcomes, better solutions, better options. . . . I'm against Obamacare, which is imposing radical change, and I would be against a conservative imposing radical change.

After a barrage of criticism from Republicans and Democrats, Congressman Ryan teamed up with Senate Democrat Ron Wyden of Oregon to develop a less radical plan. Wyden is hardly a conservative Democrat. Before coming to Congress in 1981, he cofounded Oregon's Gray Panthers, an advocacy group for seniors and retirees, and he was director of the Oregon Legal Services for the Elderly.

In the Ryan-Wyden proposal, the traditional Medicare program would remain intact so seniors could continue to have Medicare as it is now, or they could opt for a private health insurance plan. Their proposal included protections for seniors that would prevent insurance companies from denying coverage based on preexisting conditions or charging premiums based on health status, protections that are similar to those in President Obama's health care reform law.

The revised plan would give a more generous subsidy to seniors to pay the premium for a private health insurance plan. Unlike a voucher program that would give seniors a fixed amount of money to purchase health plans, the subsidy would be adjusted each year to reflect the actual cost of health insurance premiums. Still, seniors would pay the difference between the cost of insurance and the voucher or subsidy. Low-income seniors would receive a higher subsidy.

Democrat Wyden defended his position. "I will never do anything to shred or weaken it or harm [Medicare] in any way," he said. "I simply believe that there is now an opportunity for progressives and conservatives to come together and to strengthen the program for the long term and particularly deal with the costs and demographic challenges." No Democrats supported Wyden's attempt to straddle the political aisle.

Meanwhile, President Obama proposed to continue current policy that allows seniors to choose traditional Medicare or select a Medicare Advantage plan. Medicare is already on track to becoming privatized. Twenty-five percent of seniors choose a private insurance plan as an alternative to traditional Medicare.

Robert Pear wrote in the *New York Times*, "Even as President Obama accuses Mitt Romney and Representative Paul D. Ryan of trying to privatize and 'voucherize' Medicare, his administration crows about the success of private health plans in delivering . . . services to Medicare beneficiaries." Pear cites Obama administration announcements in early 2012 that Medicare Advantage premiums dropped an average of 7 percent and enrollment jumped 10 percent.

Seniors who have Medicare Advantage plans have lower out-of-pocket costs. If plans continue to have lower out-of-pocket costs, the trend toward private insurance may continue as seniors' retirement savings and income are stressed in a lackluster economy. But Medicare Advantage plans will lose some of their advantage as Medicare cuts their payments to be more on par with the amount Medicare would pay if seniors were enrolled in the traditional program. The Congressional Budget Office predicts that enrollment in Medicare Advantage plans will decline by as much as five million seniors by 2019.

Nonetheless, private health insurance companies want more boomers to enroll in their plans rather than traditional Medicare. During the health care reform debate, the health insurance industry lobbied successfully to require the uninsured to buy private insurance rather than choose a public option. The industry wants more of the Medicare market, and it will likely succeed because the money to be made is too much to resist.

Privatization has disadvantages. As more seniors enroll in Medicare Advantage plans with limited networks of doctors, they may not be able to choose any doctor they wish. Private health insurers decide the doctors and hospitals included in the provider network. In traditional Medicare, the government doesn't interfere in the patient's choice of doctor. Congressman Tom Price, a Republican from Georgia, is an orthopedic surgeon, and he tells his constituents that government bureaucrats are getting in the way of the doctor-patient relationship. In fact, insurance companies, not government bureaucrats, can get in the way of the doctor-patient relationship in privatized Medicare.

WHO WILL BEAR THE BURDEN OF CONTAINING MEDICARE SPENDING?

Both Democrats and Republicans propose to limit increases in Medicare spending. How do they propose to keep costs down? The fireworks over Medicare stem from stark differences in how the two parties answer this question. Republicans put seniors on the front lines of cost control, using free-market theories of competition and consumer choice. Democrats have a top-down approach.

Putting the Burden of Cost Control on Seniors

Republicans propose that seniors receive a subsidy, or "premium support," to defray the cost of a private health insurance plan. If a senior chooses a higher-cost plan, he or she will pay the difference. The aim, say Republicans, is to allow seniors to choose among plans and stimulate competition to keep costs in check. If costs are not controlled, seniors will bear the financial burden and pay more of their income for health care.

GOP presidential candidate Mitt Romney weighed in on the amount of subsidy while on the campaign trail in an interview with the *Washington Examiner*, saying that the growth in the subsidy will have to be limited because Medicare cannot pay an open-ended amount of money. He would let Congress determine an overall budget amount for subsidies to be appropriated each year. "And every year . . . [Congress would] pass a budget for how much the total subsidy is going to be. And that would then set the limit of how much each person is going to receive. Obviously, I've mentioned that people of lower income would get a higher subsidy than people of higher income."

Paul Ryan wants seniors to have more "skin" in the game. In fact, seniors already have plenty of "skin" in the game. Twenty-seven percent of the Social Security checks of retirees who earned modest incomes during their working life is spent on Medicare Parts B and D premiums and copayments. Higher copays might deter unnecessary doctor visits and encourage the use of less expensive generic drugs. But seniors don't have clout to negotiate favorable prices with hospitals, drug companies, or device manufacturers. Nor do they have the power to drive a poorly performing health insurer, hospital, or doctor out of business.

It may be interesting economic theory that the health care marketplace gives consumers the power to stimulate competition and lower prices. But reality doesn't match the theory. Health care is different from other goods and services. Brand-name hospitals wield enormous clout and are price setters rather than price takers. They demand and receive a high price because they can. Also, most Americans don't have the knowledge to determine the medical intervention that could yield the greatest benefit. Doctors and the health care facilities where they work are the driving force for most health care. They decide the tests, drugs, and surgeries that are rendered.

Putting the Brakes on Medicare from the Top

President Obama's plan to curtail Medicare spending was laid out in the health care reform law. An Independent Payment Advisory Board with fifteen members appointed by the president and confirmed by the Senate would recommend how to keep Medicare spending in check. They cannot fiddle with Medicare eligibility, ration care, raise premiums, or cut benefits. If Congress doesn't like the board's recommendations, it doesn't have to accept them, but it will need to propose equivalent savings to pare back Medicare spending by the same amount.

Beginning in 2014, specific spending limits will be set. If Medicare spending stays within those limits, or if Congress acts to keep Medicare spending within those bounds, the board would not need to act. Its recommendations would take effect only if Medicare spending growth is out of control and Congress fails to implement an alternative.

Lobbyists for the health care industry are vehemently opposed to the board. They claim that an unelected advisory board rather than Congress would make policy choices about Medicare. It is true that an appointed board would make recommendations to Congress. But if members of Congress don't like the proposals from the appointed board, they can substitute their own provisions to keep Medicare spending in check. The intent is to impose discipline on Congress, which has shown little capacity to restrain Medicare spending, and place the program on a sound financial footing.

Opponents allege that the board's actions will threaten the quality of health care for seniors. Yet if seniors are on the front line of controlling costs with high-deductible health plans, the quality of care can be jeopardized too.

The board can recommend additional steps, similar to those that Medicare is already taking, to stop paying hospitals and doctors for poor-quality care and unnecessary tests and surgeries that are harming seniors, not helping them. Although the board cannot change Medicare benefits, it can recommend cutting the amount of money Medicare pays drug companies and other providers who do business with Medicare if their costs are rising beyond certain levels. The industry is opposed to any action that will limit its revenue, which explains its pledge to repeal the board.

The board can recommend ramping up investigations and enforcement to curb fraud and abuse. The industry is wary of this, too, because any crackdown on white-collar fraud will uncover widespread abuses of Medicare's generosity.

Mitt Romney claimed that President Obama's approach will ration care, yet his own proposal encouraged more seniors to enroll in private plans that outsource the job of rationing to health plan company executives and managers. Medicare doesn't have enough people to police the insurers that will make these decisions. As the Medicare budget crunch hits, which it surely will, the plans will have incentive to skimp on care.

A better approach is to make the process explicit and transparent. The Independent Payment Advisory Board would do that. The perennial challenge is that elected officials don't have the gumption to rein in the excessive spending by the health care industry.

Congressman Chris Van Hollen, a Democrat from Maryland, stated the difference between the board and Ryan's "premium support" plan succinctly: "My view is that the independent board provides an important backstop to Congress for reducing the cost of Medicare without transferring risk to seniors."

Democrats are not united in their support of the board. Congressman Pete Stark, a Democrat who voted for the health care reform law, later joined with House Republicans to vote to repeal the board. Reluctant to give away power, the veteran member of Congress said, "Congress has always stepped in to strengthen Medicare's finances when needed. I have always worked on this Subcommittee to protect and strengthen Medicare and ensure it works best for its 50 million beneficiaries. . . . One only has to look at the Affordable Care Act—which extended (Medicare) solvency, slowed spending growth, lowered beneficiary costs, improved benefits, modernized our delivery system, and created new fraud-fighting tools—to see we've done a damn good job."

Still, Stark admits that the board is a far better alternative than the Ryan plan. It keeps Medicare's guaranteed benefits intact. The board cannot impose additional costs on beneficiaries or ration care. The original Ryan plan had none of these protections.

Industry and congressional opposition to the board will be hard to overcome. The Senate is required by law to confirm the fifteen members of the board, a huge hurdle. So far, the board is in limbo and is likely to remain there for a very long time.

The fight over the Independent Payment Advisory Board lays bare the battle lines in the fight for Medicare's future. On the one side are seniors, who have limited means to keep paying more. On the other side is the industry, which doesn't want any limits on how much money it can spend.

Will Obama's top-down approach control Medicare spending? One of its architects, Peter Orszag, the former White House budget director during the health care reform debate, criticized Paul Ryan's overall budget plan, including the Medicare proposal, saying it relies "on capping and punting—limiting spending to a certain level but providing no specifics on how to achieve that number." The same can be said about Obama's approach to limiting Medicare spending. It proposes a limit on spending but punts the specifics to a board that will probably never get off the ground. The question for President Obama and Democrats is how Medicare spending will be controlled without the Independent Payment Advisory Board.

WHERE DEMOCRATS AND REPUBLICANS AGREE

Beneath the sound and fury, Democratic and Republican proposals contain surprising areas of agreement. That's because there are only so many ways to put Medicare on a sound financial footing.

Both President Obama and Republicans have proposed to limit the growth in Medicare spending. In his fiscal year 2013 budget, Obama proposed holding average Medicare spending per beneficiary to GDP growth plus 0.5 percent. That same year, Paul Ryan's budget sought to similarly limit Medicare spending growth per beneficiary. So both parties have proposed to end a signature feature of Medicare, its open-ended entitlement.

Both Obama and Republicans would require higher-income seniors to pay more for Medicare. During the 2011 budget negotiations, Obama proposed raising the Medicare eligibility age from sixty-five to sixty-seven if Republicans would agree to revenue increases. Republicans have proposed increasing the retirement age too.

THE BUSINESS OF MEDICARE IS BUSINESS

During the 2012 presidential campaign, a liberal New York group, the Agenda Project, created a political attack ad aimed at Mitt Romney and Paul Ryan. In the video, a man in a dark suit who looked like Paul Ryan is pushing an old woman in a wheelchair through the woods where birds are chirping, and she is smiling. Suddenly, the pace of the walk in the woods hastens, and the older woman realizes she is being pushed to a cliff overlooking a river. The ad ends with a disturbing parting shot of granny being thrown over the cliff. It doesn't tell the public the truth about the underlying forces that are driving seniors and all Americans to the brink.

The root cause of out-of-control Medicare spending can be found in the words of President Calvin Coolidge, who said, "The business of America is business." The same is true of Medicare. The business of Medicare is business. The public is unaware of how the business of Medicare has affected virtually every aspect of care seniors receive. Thousands of American firms, large and small, rely on Medicare. They expect the program to provide them with a constant and lucrative income stream.

The dramatic growth in the number of for-profit businesses making money from Medicare is a testament to how lucrative the program is. For-profit hospitals account for 20 percent of all hospitals. Half of all hospices are now for-profit. Four out of five kidney dialysis treatment centers are for-profit.

Many health plans are still bullish on Medicare Advantage plans. Goldman Sachs calculated that for-profit health plans make $480 in profit for each Medicare beneficiary enrolled. The financial opportunities are boundless with seventy-six million boomers slated to become eligible for Medicare.

Big and small businesses push very hard to get as much money as they can from Medicare and keep it. When Medicare launched competitive bidding for wheelchairs and basic supplies such as diapers to save money, businesses protested vehemently.

Medicare had been paying "insane" rental prices to businesses for medical equipment, more than if it bought the equipment outright, according to then secretary of health and human services Michael Leavitt, who served under President George W. Bush. He gave an example in the *Wall Street Journal* of an oxygen concentrator, a device that delivers oxygen through a tube. It is used by people who have conditions such as chronic obstructive pulmonary disease that make breathing difficult. Congress writes fee schedules into the law, dictating the amount of money Medicare pays. Seniors usually rent the machines. The rental period, enshrined in law, is up to thirty-six months. The monthly rental payment, also set by law, is $198.40. The cost of renting the device for three years is $7,142. With a copay of 20 percent, seniors were paying

$1,428, which could have been used to buy two of the devices, which cost $600 each, according to Leavitt. Companies that rent the equipment help Congress write these fee schedules.

Almost five years after Congress mandated competitive bidding, Medicare conducted the first round of bidding in ten geographic areas for ten products. The bids were about 26 percent less than the amount that Medicare usually paid. As an example, the number of oxygen suppliers selected in the Greater Miami area plummeted from more than four hundred to fewer than fifty. The risk of fraud was greatly reduced because Medicare was dealing only with reputable companies. Fraud is rampant in the durable medical equipment business, having been infiltrated by organized criminal gangs in certain geographic areas. With a small number of suppliers, Medicare can keep better tabs on the firms it pays.

Two weeks after the winning bids were announced, the process was halted. Businesses slated to lose money launched an all-out lobbying campaign. Congress succumbed to the pressure and passed a law that terminated all contracts and required Medicare to rebid them.

Among the opponents of competitive bidding for wheelchairs and other supplies are people with disabilities who live in rural areas far from the companies that won the Medicare contracts. They are concerned about having little leverage against a single-source company that is unresponsive to their needs, which can pose challenges in their day-to-day life.

Almost eight years after Congress required competitive bidding, the first phase was implemented in January 2011. Once again, suppliers rallied support from members of Congress to scrap it, but this time they were unsuccessful.

SURVIVAL OF THE BIGGEST

Why is Medicare bidding for equipment and supplies, to save about a billion dollars a year, but not bidding for drugs, nor promoting competition in the market for hospital supplies, where billions of dollars in savings can be gained? The durable medical equipment business is run by many small mom-and-pop operations that don't have the political clout of multibillion-dollar corporations. The federal government picks on the easier targets. Fortune 100 companies remain unscathed in a game of survival of the biggest.

If Congress found it difficult to muster the political courage for competitive bidding for suppliers of wheelchairs and diapers, it will be far more difficult for them to make the big decisions to keep Medicare from teetering on the brink of insolvency.

Neither Democrats nor Republicans want to cut the entitlement of businesses that have failed to give Americans a fair deal. A Romney campaign aide said, "Twisting the screws on providers won't hold down costs, it just jeopardizes seniors' access to care and threatens their benefits." That's not true. Anyone who knows the inside of the health care industry can attest to rampant profligacy. The prescription for change is surgery to remove the waste while keeping benefits and access to care intact for seniors.

Neither Democrats nor Republicans have a strategy to reverse the entitlement mindset they have nurtured over many decades. During the 2012 presidential campaign, Barack Obama and Mitt Romney received campaign contributions from the health care industry to keep the spigot open. The path of least resistance is to put more burden on seniors rather than take a surgical strike at the wasteful spending. It's a game of survival of the biggest.

・ *4* ・

The Big Squeeze

$\mathscr{B}$oomers and seniors are in for a big squeeze whether Democrats or Republicans prevail in shaping Medicare's future. Medicare will become very crowded by 2030. By that time, Medicare will have added more than the current populations of Austria, Hong Kong, Israel, and Switzerland. Here is a preview of what seniors can expect.

A California nurse whose mother died of a medical error in a hospital works doubly hard at her job to keep patients safe because she doesn't want any other family to experience what her family did. A seasoned professional, she is very concerned about the quality of hospital care. During a break at work, she wrote an e-mail to us that described a typical day at her job in a medical-surgical unit of a hospital. She compared the work processes to those of a local hamburger establishment:

> In-N-Out is a fast-food hamburger chain that is always busy and very well run. The cooks slap the raw hamburger on the grill in rows very close together. The grill is always full. The cooked meat is thrown on a bun. They have to get the customers in and out quickly.
>
> In hospitals, when it comes to patients, it's all about "Get them in and get them out." They treat patients like a cheeseburger, no ketchup, no fries, no extras, we already scanned the wallet. Now get them out so you can get the ones in the ER in that bed. There is a new wallet to scan, after all. The new patient will be pushed around the grill the same way.
>
> Sometimes, well most of the time, it seems like hospitals treat patients like raw meat. From the patients' point of view, it seems as if nothing works fast and they have to wait forever. From the staff's perspective, hospital administrators make everyone take on too much

work, and as a result, patients don't get the personal attention they deserve. This affects everything—the diagnosis, the treatment, you name it. Physicians aren't listening because of time constraints or emergencies.

Patients wonder why important lab test results are overlooked or not dealt with in a timely manner, if at all. They wonder why they can't get help going to the bathroom.

Chaos erupts when a patient has more needs than your typical hamburger. If one patient starts to deteriorate and takes up all of a nurse's time, the nurse and the doctors are pushed to the limit. All patients are individuals, not hamburgers, and the wrenches start flying.

Doctors are being asked to see more and more patients. After a while, the stress can be unbelievable. You don't care anymore. You can't spend enough time with a patient and you feel trapped in the system. The good doctors are evaporating as they crank out widgets.

There's the old song from Burger King: "Hold the pickles, hold the lettuce, special orders don't upset us." Burger King wants you to come back. A hospital doesn't have to be good to patients because if they get sick someday, they may have no choice but to come back.

This description reveals the impact of industrialization in health care, the process by which traditionally nonindustrial sectors such as health care become increasingly similar to the manufacturing sector of the economy.

The industrial model excels at producing commodities efficiently whether they are smartphones, cars, or houses. As health care has taken on characteristics of the industrial model, health care services are being treated as if they were a commodity. A commodity is a good or service whose wide availability and similarity reduce the decision about buying it to price. If only the healing of the human body were that simple.

The mainstream business media touts the trend toward health care as a commodity as progress, a coming of age. Dr. Ralph de la Torre is a former chief of cardiac surgery at Beth Israel Deaconess Medical Center in Boston and now CEO of Boston-based Steward Health Care, a for-profit hospital system that buys community hospitals. It is owned by private investment firm Cerberus Capital Management, named for the three-headed hound in Greek mythology that is guarding the gates of the underworld. In an interview in *Fortune*, de la Torre said,

You have to look back at America and the trends in industries that have gone from being art to science, to being commodities. Health care is becoming a commodity. The car industry started off as an art, people hand-shaping the bodies, hand-building the engines. As it became a commodity and was all about making cars accessible to everybody, it became more about standardization. It's not different from the banking industry and other industries as they've matured. Health care is finally maturing as an industry. . . . It's getting economies of scale and in many ways making it a commodity.

Where does the mindset of health care as a commodity come from? Companies that sell commodities such as CT scanners, antibiotics, and hip implants are a likely source. For them, commodities are valued because they are a source of revenue. The work in health care today of prescribing and administering drugs, using equipment, and implanting devices brings monetary value to companies that manufacture them. So that is what doctors and nurses do. Time spent talking to a patient provides no monetary value to any health care businesses. Hence, it is weeded out from day-to-day work. The industrial model is successfully engineering communication between patients and their doctors and nurses out of the system. It is also engineering out of the system essential communication among doctors, nurses, and other health care professionals.

The industrial model explains why television medical dramas no longer feature primary-care physicians like Dr. Marcus Welby, who talked to his patients, and instead feature doctors such as the irascible Dr. House, who performs every imaging scan and test known to human kind. Viewers' minds are marinated to believe this is good medicine. Manufacturers of imaging equipment are acknowledged in the credits at the end of the program.

The mindset of health care as a commodity ignores the unique physiology and medical history of each person. Two people can have an entirely different physical response to the same medical intervention. Commodification of health care cripples the ability of the health care system—and the doctors and nurses who take care of patients—to respond to the unique and variable needs of people who are sick. Nothing can be further from the reality of what it takes to heal a human body than the treatment of patients as interchangeable parts.

Commodification runs roughshod over science and evidence of what works in medicine. It ignores a patient's preferences and beliefs about the value of an elective surgery or test. The system is set up to sell them, so that is what the system does and that's what patients get, whether they want them or not. As hospitals spend more of their budgets on equipment, drugs, and supplies to deliver commodities, nursing staff are cut to levels that can make it impossible for them to care for patients safely.

Industrialization assumes that people who provide health care services are interchangeable parts, when, in fact, enormous variation exists in the knowledge, skill, and competence of doctors, nurses, and all other health care professionals.

Standardization of the process of work in health care delivery systems is different from commodification and can make an essential contribution to quality and safety. Checklists used to prevent hospital-acquired infections are an example of standardization of work. So is the "time-out" prior to surgery where the surgical team verifies the patient's identity, the purpose of the surgery, and the part of the body that will be operated on. Standardization of work processes brings a rigor and precision to a highly complex process fraught with opportunity for human error, which we wrote about in our book *Wall of Silence*.

Because of the industrial model, seniors, boomers, and everyone else will see their health care become more depersonalized and a source of dissatisfaction. Health care is being driven by an intention that is business-minded and has nothing to do with understanding the intricate ways in which the body heals, nor how it can be so easily harmed by treatment carried out when dollar signs are the driving force behind it.

Industrialization and its demands for high productivity are a cause of widespread doctor burnout and unhappiness. Researchers from the Mayo Clinic surveyed more than seven thousand doctors, and an alarming number of them—46 percent—had at least one symptom of burnout. They reported being emotionally exhausted or having feelings of depersonalization. Doctors were more burned-out than the general working population and more unhappy with their work–life balance. In the coming years, stress will increase as doctors are required to see more patients as boomers age and more newly insured people use more health care services.

The industrialization and commodification of health care are driving out the humanitarian and scientific roots of medical practice. As these underpinnings are sidelined and drowned out by the commercial imperative, health care will cease to be the humanitarian and scientific enterprise it is meant to be.

DOES YOUR DOCTOR ACCEPT MEDICARE?

If you are a boomer and think your doctor will continue to be your doctor when you are on Medicare, you might want to check to be certain. A woman we know had been going to her doctor at Northwestern Memorial Hospital Women's Group in Chicago for several years for regular checkups. She liked her doctor, so when she turned sixty-five, she called to make an appointment as usual. The office staff said that the practice does not accept Medicare. The practice website confirms this policy. "I was so stunned that this premier group of doctors doesn't accept Medicare," the patient said. "It never dawned on me that it would be a problem."

The office staff offered her the option to pay $250 in cash for the annual exam. She declined because she was concerned about the cost if something unexpected was found and required a major expense. After calling four other doctors' offices and learning they didn't accept Medicare, she went on the Internet and found an excellent practice where she now receives her care.

A local television station in North Carolina teamed up with AARP volunteers to be secret shoppers. They called family doctors' offices to ask if the doctors are accepting new Medicare patients. In the Triangle area of Raleigh, Durham, and Chapel Hill, the volunteers discovered that seniors can have a hard time finding a doctor. Nearly 50 percent of the two hundred doctors they called were not taking new Medicare patients. Among those who were, many require seniors to pay the doctor directly and file Medicare forms to be reimbursed. Although this cuts down on the paperwork for the doctor's office, it places the onus on seniors, who may have difficulty coping with mountains of paperwork.

The local news station reported that it contacted Medicare program officials and learned that the agency was planning its own secret shopper investigation, but the plan was derailed after opposition from doctors.

The official stance from Medicare is that 98 percent of doctors in North Carolina have agreed to participate in the program, but as the secret shoppers learned, the reality is far different from what the federal government tells seniors. If Medicare cannot be honest with seniors about this basic fact, what else is Medicare not telling seniors?

HOLES IN THE CHEESE

Whether Democrats or Republicans prevail in shaping Medicare's future, the program will be expected to take care of a much larger family with a budget that will be squeezed.

These changes will be little different than the changes employees with private health insurance are experiencing. As the average cost of an employer-based health insurance policy climbed to $15,745 in 2012, employers are tightening their purse strings. As costs continue to rise, employees have insurance with skimpier coverage and higher premiums, deductibles, and copayments. Even those with private health insurance say that cost has become more of an impediment to care, according to the Center for Studying Health System Change, a Washington, DC, health care policy analysis group. Medicare will not be immune to these trends.

In the coming decades, health care will become more like airline travel, where first-class passengers are treated to private suites and three-star meals. Economy-class passengers are packed in like sardines and pay extra for food, checked bags, and more legroom. Whether Democrats or Republicans prevail in determining Medicare's future, seniors and boomers will have to fasten their seat belts and hang on in their middle seats during the turbulent ride that lies ahead.

Part II

WHERE YOUR MONEY GOES: THE BUSINESS OF MEDICARE

In part II we go behind the scenes and take a look at the business of Medicare to shine a light on where your money goes, who gets it, and how they get it. As you will see, the business of Medicare is like no other.

Chapter 5 tells the true story of Mr. Davis, who lives in the rolling hills of rural Somerset, Kentucky. He wrote a letter to the editor of his local newspaper about a $244,000 bill he received from a local hospital for a procedure and a one-night stay. We take a look at a hospital in the community, its parent company, and its corporate financial strategy to understand why a hospital bill can be so costly. Mr. Davis's story is a microcosm for all of Medicare and is repeated every day across America.

Chapter 6 examines the business of Medicare billing and how hospitals and other health care facilities work intently to submit bills for as many tests and treatments as possible, at the highest rate possible. We take a close look at consulting and marketing firms whose sole purpose is to advise health care providers on how to take full advantage of Medicare's loopholes.

Medicare was designed without any red lights to stop excessive profiteering at taxpayer and seniors' expense. In chapter 7 we reveal how Medicare officials are barred by laws written with the help of industry lobbyists from being good stewards of the public's money. We show how Medicare pays for drugs, doctor visits, and Medicare Advantage plans in the most expensive way imaginable.

When a Night in the Hospital
Costs More Than a House

$\mathcal{N}$estled in the Appalachian Mountains in Kentucky, Pulaski County is dry, mostly. It is home to Sinking Valley Vineyards, whose specialty is a sweet red wine with collector labels that depict the beginning, enforcement, and repeal of prohibition. The county seat is in the town of Somerset, the home of Kingsford charcoal briquettes, which fire up grills for countless Memorial Day barbeques, and Duraflame logs, which warm fireplaces in homes around the country.

A property in the town of Somerset was listed for sale on the real estate website Trulia. The address was Medicare Drive, Somerset, Kentucky 42501. Medicare has no plans to move its offices from its headquarters in Baltimore, Maryland. More likely, the street was a place whose businesses were counting on Medicare to fill their coffers.

A photo accompanying the listing showed undeveloped land with buildings in the background. The price tag was $1.5 million, and the property description read as follows:

> This tract of land was originally developed for medical/professional facilities. It offers easy convenience to the hospital, easy access to all of Somerset's main highways; the property has been developed with paved roads, underground utilities, and is on city sewer. The 20 lots can be bought individually from $99K up to $199K. If the entire development were to be purchased it could be a great investment for any investor.

The listing stood out from the 189 homes advertised for sale in Somerset whose average price was $209,000. A modest ranch on West

Bourbon Road with four bedrooms and two baths on one-third of an acre was listed for $99,900. A four-bedroom house on Windy Hills Drive with three baths and four acres of land could be bought for $249,000. Advertised as "heaven on earth," it had four thousand square feet of space, two complete kitchen setups with appliances, and two family rooms and fireplaces.

Underneath the veneer of heaven on earth is the reality of life. The local Somerset newspaper, the *Commonwealth Journal*, published a letter to the editor penned by Mr. Davis, a resident of the town. He fumed about a hospital bill he received after being admitted overnight for an unspecified procedure. He wrote, "I needed to have a relatively minor procedure performed. This procedure required an operating room, supporting staff, the implantation of a medical device, and a one-night stay in the facility for observation. . . . The bill that I received from this facility was in the amount of $244,000 plus." That amount for a one-night stay in the hospital is the cost of a nice house in Somerset, bought free and clear without a mortgage.

Fortunately for Mr. Davis, he had Medicare and supplemental insurance coverage. He wondered what would have happened if he had been uninsured, so he called the hospital and spoke to a person in the billing office who confirmed that the hospital would seek full payment if he lacked insurance. In the letter to the local newspaper, he wrote that he could have been "left destitute as the result of just one huge medical bill from a for-profit facility. . . . If I had not had Medicare in its present form, it is obvious that this facility would have aggressively pursued payment of the $244,000 amount."

Fortunately for taxpayers, Medicare and his supplemental insurance authorized payment of just over $18,000 for his one-night stay in the hospital to cover the bill in full. The hospital accepted it under its terms of participation in Medicare. Mr. Davis said the physician who performed the procedure charged a reasonable fee, but the hospital needed to be constrained. Mr. Davis is a polite gentleman and didn't mention the name of the hospital.

Mr. Davis's letter was prompted by an article in the *Commonwealth Journal* written by a local columnist, Richard Moore, who commented about the poor-quality care in Somerset. "There is widespread discontent with Lake Cumberland Regional Medical Center about its quality, pricing and customer service," Moore wrote. "It is my experience and my opinion that for most serious medical problems, better service can be obtained in Lexington, Louisville or Nashville for equal or less money." He asked local readers to submit letters about their experience with the hospital.

The only for-profit hospital within miles of Somerset is Lake Cumberland Regional Hospital. The buildings in the picture on the real estate website were those of the hospital. It is owned by LifePoint, a Brentwood, Tennessee, company that owns fifty-four hospitals located mostly in the southeastern part of the country. The company's stock is publicly traded on the NASDAQ.

When the chief financial officer of LifePoint, Jeff Sherman, presented at a JP Morgan Healthcare Conference in San Francisco, he laid out the company's strategy. "In 51 of our 54 markets, we are the only hospital in the community," Sherman told conference participants. "This gives us negotiating advantage when we negotiate our rates."

A company report filed with the Securities and Exchange Commission punctuated the point, saying, "We believe that non-urban healthcare markets are attractive because non-urban communities have smaller populations, they generally have fewer hospitals and other healthcare service providers. Additionally, because non-urban hospitals are generally sole providers or one of a small group of providers in their markets, there is limited competition."

ARE YOU GETTING WHAT YOU PAY FOR?

The same month that Mr. Davis wrote his letter to the newspaper, a report on the quality of care in Lake Cumberland Regional Hospital was posted on the website of The Joint Commission, the Chicago-based group that inspects and accredits many hospitals around the country. Medicare requires that hospitals be accredited by The Joint Commission or other designated entity to be eligible to receive payment. Accreditation standards cover a range of topics, from ensuring fire safety to preventing prescription drug errors and hospital-acquired infections.

In June 2011, surveyors from The Joint Commission who inspected the hospital found that it was not in compliance with important standards that every hospital is expected to meet. The Joint Commission posted the list of standards the hospital did not meet on its website. They included the following:

- Maintain proper medical records: Hospitals are required to maintain complete and accurate medical records for each individual patient. They should contain information that reflects the patient's care, surgeries and other high-risk procedures, and follow-up care.
- Take action to prevent medical mistakes and infections: Hospitals must implement standard patient-safety procedures to prevent hospital-acquired infections, eliminate blood transfusion errors so patients receive blood that is the appropriate type, prevent medication errors involving drugs that look alike and whose names sound alike, ensure doctors and nurses do a "time-out" before a surgery to verify the patient's identity and the correct site of the procedure to prevent wrong-site and wrong-person surgeries, and allow any doctor, nurse, or other person who provides care to report concerns about safety or the quality of care to The Joint Commission without retaliation by the hospital.
- Ensure accountability for patient care: Doctors in the hospital are required to oversee the quality of patient care, treatment, and services provided by practitioners who have hospital privileges to admit patients. Medical staff bylaws must address self-governance and accountability to the hospital's governing body. The hospital's governing body is ultimately accountable for the safety and quality of care, treatment, and services.
- Provide care properly: The hospital is required to assess and reassess patients on a regular basis. The hospital is also required to provide care, treatment, and services as ordered or prescribed, and in accordance with law and regulation. It must render care to the patient before initiating operative or other high-risk procedures, including those that require the administration of moderate or deep sedation or anesthesia.
- Ensure building and fire safety: Hospitals are required to maintain a safe, functional environment, which includes maintaining fire-safety equipment and systems to extinguish fires. They must also protect patients during periods of construction of new hospital buildings nearby.

The Joint Commission does not publicly report the specific circumstances surrounding the deficiencies. Surveyors returned to the hospital to determine if the deficiencies had been corrected. Four months later, a new report on The Joint Commission website stated that the hospital is fully accredited.

Most hospitals accredited by The Joint Commission are listed on its website as fully accredited. Lake Cumberland Regional Hospital is one of a small percentage of hospitals that was, for a short time, reported as needing improvement. The Joint Commission rarely revokes a hospital's accreditation.

Jeff Sherman, the LifePoint chief financial officer, said to the JP Morgan conference attendees that the hospital company is aggressively recruiting physicians to work in its hospitals. Without doctors, hospitals cannot make money and meet shareholders' demands for a solid return on their investment.

Sherman explained that his company is targeting a 3 to 5 percent increase in earnings per share for its stock in the next several years. The only way that a hospital can continually increase profitability is to increase revenue and decrease expenses. Hospitals increase revenue by admitting more patients, billing more services per patient, and increasing the amount of money it bills for each service. Hospitals typically cut expenses by reducing the number of nurses and hiring nurses with lower skill levels.

LifePoint has a checkered lineage. In 1999 it spun off from Columbia-HCA, which is the for-profit hospital company that paid 1.7 billion dollars in fines and penalties in 2000 and 2003 in what was then the largest federal fraud settlement in U.S. history. FBI agents searched Columbia-HCA facilities and found that it overcharged and fraudulently billed Medicare, inflated the seriousness of diagnoses to make more money, and paid kickbacks to doctors for referring patients to the company's hospitals, among other offenses. The company pleaded guilty to fourteen felonies and paid the fines. Now called HCA, it was founded by the father of former U.S. senator Bill Frist, a Republican from Tennessee who was in office while the investigation was taking place. LifePoint took over the smaller community hospitals that Columbia-HCA no longer wanted.

WHEN THE PRICE IS WRONG

If Mr. Davis had gone to a different hospital, he may have been charged a much lower price. Enormous variation exists in how much hospitals charge for the exact same procedure.

When Dr. Renee Hsia at the University of California at San Francisco studied the charges for more than nineteen thousand cases of acute appendicitis performed in California hospitals, she and her team found huge differences, ranging from $1,529 to $182,955. For the study, only those who had no complications and were hospitalized up to three days were included.

Hospitals with the highest charges were not rare, with many billing more than $100,000. Many hospitals also charged relatively modest amounts. Hospitals can charge whatever they want because there are no rules for how much they can charge. No market mechanism or government regulatory authority prohibits price gouging.

The median charge for treating acute appendicitis from a county public hospital was 36.6 percent lower than a nonprofit hospital. For-profit hospitals charged the highest amount.

The variation in charges is only part of the challenge that patients encounter. Hsia and her team found that the median charge for treating acute appendicitis was $33,611, an amount they said "should alarm those making decisions about our society's ability to obtain medical care without financial catastrophe." If a person has the misfortune of experiencing acute appendicitis in California it could cost more than half the annual median household income in the state, which is $60,883.

Pricey hospital bills drive up the cost of medical care for everyone. All across America, as people spend money on expensive medical care, they have less money to spend in the grocery store and restaurants or give to their place of worship and local charities. The federal government has less money to fix crumbling roads and bridges. States have less money to pay teachers' pensions. Taxpayers pay higher property taxes to cover the cost of health care for public employees who fight fires, teach their children, and maintain roads and other essential services.

High profits in health care attract more investors, who underwrite the construction of yet more hospitals that, in turn, charge out-of-sight prices.

To bring more openness to the prices that hospitals charge, New York–based FAIR Health is an independent nonprofit that has a national database of billions of billed medical services. It gives consumers free information about charges for common tests and procedures in their zip code and how much insurers pay for an out-of-network provider. The cost of a basic colonoscopy, for instance, in a suburban community in Long Island is $1,299. Not all medical procedures and tests are listed. There are gaps in price information for surgeries such as angioplasty or back surgery. Nonetheless, it is a needed start to price transparency.

When a person is writhing in agony from acute appendicitis, it is not the time to go online and find the hospital with the lowest price. The Latin word for patient means "to suffer." In the middle of agony, people will pay almost anything to stop the pain.

Proponents of more consumer choice and competition believe that health insurance has insulated people from the true cost, so they use more tests, services, and drugs. It is true that people are far less sensitive to cost when they are not paying the full bill. When treatment is not urgent, the use of the emergency room for a cold or cough is wasteful use.

Chief proponent of consumer choice and competition Paul Ryan said, "When we pay directly for something, and we know how much it costs, we have a strong incentive to demand the best value. In health care, we don't. Is it any wonder that the costs keep rising?"

Times have changed since consumer choice and competition were first introduced more than thirty years ago. Today, profiteering in health care has become the norm and a major reason that costs keep rising. In Somerset, Mr. Davis had zero negotiating power with the hospital.

Price isn't everything. To know the price of everything without knowing its value has little meaning. We met a state legislator from the East Coast who heard one of us speak about the pervasive overtreatment in health care. He said that when he goes to his doctor every three months, he gets a chest X-ray every time. When asked if he had an underlying medical condition, he said he didn't. He began to wonder whether they are really necessary. X-rays emit radiation, so if they are not needed, it's best to avoid them. The legislator vowed to ask his doctor if they are medically necessary. Even if a medical test or procedure is less expensive at one hospital, it is no bargain if it is not warranted. The best care is only the care you need, not the care you don't.

Back in Somerset, the real estate firm that listed the property on Medicare Drive had erred, we learned later. The actual name of the street is Medcare Drive. No matter the name, if the hospital can charge patients enormous sums, it will be paved with the money of people of modest means from their Social Security checks and life savings.

As for the $18,000 payment that Medicare and supplemental insurance made for Mr. Davis's one-night stay in the hospital, it is still a lot of money. It is about 70 percent of the median household income in Somerset, which is $26,000.

Americans don't mind when people get rich. Nor do they mind free enterprise. Americans believe that money should be made fairly, not by taking advantage of people with modest means. The chasm between those who unduly profit from health care and those who pay for it is wide already. In the future, the chasm will widen more because there is nothing to stop it. Too often, people who work in health care have become disconnected from the people they are supposed to serve. Sick people are a means to an end rather than the purpose of health care.

This is what happens as the business of Medicare extends its grip on the people living in the gently rolling hills across America.

· 6 ·

Bill, Baby, Bill

$\mathcal{W}$hen the sun shines brightly on the Himalayas in the northern part of the Indian subcontinent, shadows constantly shift as the angle of the light changes every nanosecond. The sun brings needed warmth at high elevations where hardy residents of the steep valleys have one of the highest rates of cataracts in the world.

A cataract is a clouding of the lens in the eye that is the leading cause of blindness in the world. Seniors become dependent on their family and neighbors to do basic tasks they once performed independently for decades. They can no longer farm their lands, herd their animals, or walk to fetch water. Medical care is far away and few doctors are available to help amid the mountainous beauty.

Thousands of miles away in the United States, by age eighty more than half of Americans either have a cataract or have had cataract surgery to remove the cloudy lens and replace it with an artificial one to restore sight. Medicare makes cataract surgery possible for millions of seniors every year. Restoring sight is a gift that keeps on giving.

This is the purpose of Medicare, to make life better by lightening the burdens that accompany an aging body. This is the Medicare that most seniors know. There is another side to Medicare that most people don't know: the business of Medicare billing.

The business of Medicare is unlike any other business. Hospital executives can build new facilities and buy expensive new equipment knowing they have a steady revenue source from Medicare and private insurers.

In December 1992, 883 hospitals in the United States had heart bypass surgery centers. During the next ten years, hospitals built 301 more, a 34 percent increase. Most of the new centers were located in the eastern part of the United States and the Midwest, with many concentrated in the mid-Atlantic region. More than 80 percent of Americans lived within thirty miles of an existing one before the expansion. After the expansion, travel time for seniors to the nearest cardiac surgery program changed little. Duplicative facilities had been built, and access did not improve for those who might need the procedure. The dramatic increase in the number of facilities occurred when the number of heart bypass surgeries performed nationally was declining.

Here is another example. In 2001, 1,176 hospitals of the almost 5,000 were equipped to perform angioplasty, a procedure to open up clogged arteries in the heart. Nearly 80 percent of people in America lived within an hour's drive to one of these hospitals. By 2006, another 519 hospitals spent patients' money to equip their facilities to perform angioplasty. Yet the enormous sums that were spent did not increase access for more people. Instead, the additional capacity was built in areas where people already had access to treatment.

Hospital executives are not paid to be good stewards of Medicare's resources. They are paid to do the exact opposite, which is to maximize revenue. They bear little personal risk if investments fail because hospitals are rarely allowed to go out of business. They can raid Medicare's larder and leave it to seniors and taxpayers to replenish it. This is the face of Medicare that most people do not see.

THE OTHER MORAL HAZARD IN HEALTH CARE

Moral hazard became a popular term in the national dialogue after the 2008 banking crisis nearly brought the country to its knees. Reckless behavior by banks caused the near collapse of the financial sector, and millions of people lost their jobs and their homes in the mortgage meltdown. The banks knew that the federal government would bail them out if they gambled away other peoples' money, and it did. Taxpayers were irate at the prospect of the seven-hundred-billion-dollar bailout in 2009 that went to the same people who put their own financial self-interest above that of their customers. In a classic case of moral hazard, the bailout rewarded bad behavior. Bank executives paid themselves multimillion-dollar bonuses, a reward for breaking the rules that society needs to function.

In health care, moral hazard usually refers to people who use more health care services because they have insurance and don't pay the full cost themselves. Critics of Medicare such as conservative economist Walter Williams say that insurance creates moral hazard because seniors are less motivated to take care of themselves when others pay part of the bill. The antidote, insurance critics say, is for the insured to have more "skin in the game" and pay more, a theme that Congressman Paul Ryan uses to bolster his idea of "premium support" for Medicare.

Moral hazard is hardly ever discussed when it involves hospital executives, shareholders of for-profit facilities, and doctors, who can bill Medicare, private insurers, and everyone else and waste other peoples' money on excess capacity.

Scottish philosopher, Adam Smith, author of the 1776 treatise *The Wealth of Nations*, bluntly stated the motivation that companies and managers have to be profligate with other peoples' money when they have no "skin" in the game:

> The directors of such companies . . . being the managers of other people's money rather than their own, it cannot well be expected that they should watch over it with the same anxious vigilance. . . . Negligence and profusion must always prevail, more or less, in the management of such a company.

With so much duplication of facilities, where do the hospitals find patients to fill up the new facilities? Most observers might assume that people in the community need the treatments that hospitals can now perform. Otherwise, why would hospitals build the extra capacity?

THE MOTHER OF ALL MORAL HAZARD

Many hospitals that build excess capacity use it to treat people who should not be treated, the ultimate in moral hazard. In August 2012, the *New York Times* reported that HCA, the largest for-profit hospital chain in the United States with 163 hospitals, had evidence that cardiologists at its facilities were performing unnecessary cardiac procedures. The *Times* had access to thousands of pages of e-mails from company executives, confidential memos, transcripts from hearings, and reports from outside experts about the medical necessity of the procedures.

At an HCA-owned hospital in Lawnwood, Florida, 1,200 cardiac catheterizations were determined to be medically unnecessary according to a confidential internal review conducted by the hospital. During a cardiac catheterization, a small, thin tube is placed in a blood vessel and travels up to the arteries surrounding the heart. If the arteries are blocked, an angioplasty can be performed in which a small balloon is inflated to open up the blockage and allow blood to flow. A small, stainless tube called a stent might be placed to prop open the artery.

Another HCA hospital, Regional Medical Center Bayonet Point in Hudson, Florida, performed about 150 angioplasty procedures that were deemed medically inappropriate. There was an epidemic of stents, too.

An external review of medical records conducted by a firm at the request of HCA found that physicians overstated the extent of blockages in arteries, sometimes by as much as 80 to 90 percent, when, upon closer scrutiny, the blockages were much less significant and below the threshold for intervention.

Patients were harmed. In one case, a woman with no significant heart disease went into cardiac arrest after a blood vessel was perforated during an unnecessary procedure to insert a stent. She was in the hospital for several days. Implanting a stent is not risk free and can cause a heart attack, a breakdown in the lining of the artery, or cuts to the artery.

Although some of the doctors were accused in internal documents of performing unnecessary procedures, they continued to practice at HCA hospitals. The doctors deny they provided unnecessary treatment.

WHEN MEDICARE TRIES TO CRACK DOWN

A cardiac defibrillator implanted in the chest acts as a small generator that delivers an electrical jolt if a potentially life-threatening heart rhythm occurs. Defibrillators can prevent sudden cardiac death in some people. In 2005 Medicare began to reimburse hospitals and doctors for implanting them.

As with many good ideas in medicine, cardiac defibrillators have been misused. Doctors have implanted the devices in people for whom it causes more harm than good, according to a study published in the *Journal of the American Medical Association*. Of the more than one hundred thousand people who had defibrillators implanted from 2006 to 2009, 22.5 percent, or more than one in five, should not have had the procedure. They suffered from more life-threatening complications. Certain hospitals had especially high rates—40 percent or more—of inappropriate use of defibrillators.

The public is not permitted to know which hospitals had the highest inappropriate use, nor the doctors who misused the devices. Typically, they are not named because the hospital industry and the American Medical Association don't want the information to be made public. The study was funded by the National Institutes of Health and paid for by taxpayers. Medicare has been paying for those medically inappropriate procedures, and here's what happened when it tried to stop.

Medicare officials announced a crackdown in late 2011 on doctors and hospitals with a high rate of improper payments. Medicare defines improper payments as those that include coding errors and mistakes in calculating payment. Improper payments also include payments for procedures performed without adequate documentation of medical necessity. Improper payments are not considered fraud, which is a separate category and requires evidence of intent to defraud Medicare. In 2010 Medicare reported it made forty-eight billion dollars in improper payments.

The probe was targeted at eleven states: Florida, California, Michigan, Texas, New York, Louisiana, Illinois, Pennsylvania, Ohio, North Carolina, and Missouri. In Florida, Medicare planned a review of 100 percent of all claims for fifteen procedures known to be widely used inappropriately, including implanted cardiac defibrillators, cardiac stents, heart bypass surgery, and back surgery. A smaller percentage of claims were slated for review in the other states.

Hospital payments would be withheld for these procedures until after all the patients' medical records were reviewed by independent doctors for medical necessity, which would be complete within sixty days. Doctors would continue to be paid pending the review. If the review found that a procedure the doctor billed for was not medically necessary, the hospital's claim would be denied and the doctor would receive a "take back" letter stating that the improper payments had to be returned.

Florida was the first state targeted for the audit because of its track record of high levels of improper payments. Doctors employed by regional contractors hired by Medicare would perform the reviews, not Medicare employees.

The Florida chapter of the American College of Cardiology and its cardiologist members vowed to fight back. In a letter to members, it explained Medicare's justification for the audit, saying that Medicare believes that 50 percent or more of cardiac procedures done on inpatients are unjustified on the basis of available hospital documentation. In some cases, the error rate is felt to be as high as 100 percent. "This estimate apparently arises from White House and Congressional concerns that unnecessary procedures are being funded," it told its members. The error rates are based on testing of medical records against the requirements that doctors have to meet to justify Medicare coverage and payment. The cardiologists vowed to fight back against what it perceived to be government intrusion.

Business news reporters were the first to break the story. *Bloomberg News* reported that a Wells Fargo analyst issued a report for investors that described Medicare's planned actions and cited "reimbursement experts who have all indicated that this initiative seems onerous for hospitals and will likely reduce procedure volume because hospitals will begin making sure that every patient meets the coverage criteria."

Wall Street didn't welcome the news. *Forbes* reported strong reactions in the market. Stock prices of for-profit hospital chain Tenet dropped 11 percent, and device manufacturer Medtronic lost 6 percent of its stock value.

The cardiologists asserted they would be "threatened" by unjustified government action. For them, the battle was about money. No acknowledgment or concern was expressed for seniors who may have been harmed by inappropriate medical care and paid substantial sums out of pocket unnecessarily.

Public interest advocates are too few in number to have entered the fray. Patients have no voice or representation in the back-and-forth battle between government and the doctors and hospitals. They bear the greatest burden when surgery is performed that is medically unjustified.

Bowing to the pressure, six weeks later Medicare announced that it postponed its plan to review possible improper medical care provided to seniors. Although Medicare tried to be a good steward of its resources, it was stopped in its tracks. The audit eventually started, but opposition has been fierce.

In a broadside against Medicare's move, the American Medical Association wrote a letter to Medicare officials requesting that the claims review plan be rescinded altogether, claiming that seniors' access to care would be placed at risk because doctors and hospitals would be reluctant to treat patients while under such scrutiny and the threat of nonpayment. Seven months later, the American Hospital Association weighed in with a lawsuit against Medicare claiming that Medicare auditors are denying hospitals money for medically necessary care. The federal government is not giving up. HCA revealed in a filing with the Securities and Exchange Commission in August 2012 that U.S. Department of Justice prosecutors are reviewing the billing and medical records at 95 of its 163 hospitals for appropriate use of implantable defibrillators. Irrespective of the outcome of the investigation, one certainty is that federal prosecutors will have full employment in the coming years as the health care industry continues to bend and break the rules.

CHOOSING WISELY

In the spirit of making health care better, doctors from nine specialties and *Consumer Reports*, the leading nonprofit independent consumer organization, launched an initiative called Choosing Wisely in the spring of 2012. Its purpose is to reduce the use of unnecessary tests and treatments that many Americans receive.

Each group of specialists prepared a list of "Five Things Physicians and Patients Should Question" that is meant to stimulate discussion about the need for many frequently ordered tests and treatments. They are overused and can cause more harm than good. Millions of seniors and the Medicare program are paying for them. Also, they consume a lot of time and cause unnecessary worry.

The Choosing Wisely campaign appealed to doctors' sense of professionalism and urged them to be good stewards of the public's resources. Most health care spending begins with the doctor's pen or computer keystroke that triggers a cascade of tests, drugs, and procedures. Here are examples of tests and procedures identified in the Choosing Wisely campaign that are performed too frequently:

Electrocardiograms (EKGs) and other heart-screening tests. Heart-screening tests can be lifesaving for people with chest pain or other symptoms of heart disease. The American College of Cardiology does not recommend that people with no symptoms and who are at low risk for heart disease have a routine EKG, which tests the electrical activity of the heart, nor should they have a cardiac stress or treadmill test that checks for blockages in the arteries. But a 2010 *Consumer Reports* survey found that 44 percent of people with no signs of heart disease had an EKG, exercise stress test, or ultrasound. Doctors say that this practice can lead to unnecessary invasive procedures and excess radiation exposure without providing a benefit. The results are far more likely to show a false positive, which can lead to more unnecessary tests and risky heart procedures rather than find a real problem.

Brain imaging tests for common headaches. Doctors at the American College of Radiology say that CT scans and MRIs for common headaches are not necessary. But they are performed frequently. The risk of these tests is that they will reveal an image that looks to be a problem but is not. For example, a test result showing what may look like a brain aneurysm might be simply a harmless twist in a blood vessel. More doctor appointments and tests will be needed to find out, causing unnecessary worry. Unless a headache is accompanied by symptoms such as a fever or vomiting, or blurred speech or vision, imaging tests for common headaches can be avoided, and so can the dose of radiation that comes from a CT scan.

Colonoscopy to check for cancer. Many boomers and seniors on Medicare are being given colonoscopies too frequently. That is the conclusion drawn by the American Gastroenterological Association, which says that colorectal cancer screening is needed only every ten years for people without any increased risk such as family history of the disease. The procedure itself has risks, namely, perforation of the colon and adverse reactions to the anesthesia, which, while rare, are real.

Bone scans to check for osteoporosis in women. Doctors are performing bone density tests called DXA scans on women beginning at age fifty, even if they don't have any risk factors. This is not considered good medical practice, according to the American Academy of Family Physicians. The scans involve X-rays of the hip, for instance, to determine the concentration of calcium and other minerals in the bone. Test results can prompt doctors to prescribe unnecessary drugs that have serious side effects. Women should wait until at least age sixty-five, unless they have risks such as low body weight and have smoked.

Antibiotics and CT scans for sinus infections. Most sinus infections are caused by viruses, and antibiotics are ineffective. They won't relieve symptoms nor spur recovery. Most sinus infections resolve without treatment in two weeks. Nonetheless, doctors prescribe the drugs for 80 percent of people who come to them with sinus infections. The immense overuse of antibiotics is causing the mutation of bacteria that have become resistant to the arsenal of drugs. If antibiotics are taken unnecessarily, they may not be effective when they are really needed to combat a bacterial infection.

Allergy testing. About thirty-five million Americans have seasonal allergies, and millions more believe they are allergic to certain foods. Some doctors and other health providers now perform a blood test for food allergies. But doctors from the American Academy of Allergy Asthma & Immunology say some tests are not useful. For seasonal allergies, many doctors run a slew of skin and blood tests that are not necessary. Instead, a few specific tests when symptoms occur is a better approach. Fewer tests can reduce unnecessary use of allergy drugs.

Over-the-counter and other painkillers. Many people with heart and kidney disease use over-the-counter Advil, Motrin (ibuprofen), or prescriptions such as Celebrex when they have joint pain or a headache. These drugs can be dangerous when people with high blood pressure take them. They raise blood pressure and can interfere with kidney function.

X-ray, CT scan, or MRI for low back pain. Most people who have low back pain get better in four to six weeks whether or not they go to the doctor. If older people get an imaging test, experts say the results will almost always show an incidental finding that has nothing to do with the back pain and could lead to more unwarranted tests and possibly back surgery. Often the body can heal itself, but it has to be given a chance.

The Choosing Wisely campaign is appealing to doctors who have a patient's best interests at heart. For doctors for whom private gain is more important than the well-being of patients, the Choosing Wisely campaign will not resonate. For them, medicine is a business rather than a profession. As a seasoned physician said at a private dinner, "There are three kinds of doctors: those who are in it for the right reasons, those who are in it for the money, and those who are watching to see who wins."

Choosing Wisely is antithetical to the companies that sell CT scanners, MRI machines, treadmills, and the antibiotics and allergy drugs used to provide unnecessary and inappropriate testing and treatment. Their aim is to sell more, not choose wisely.

MEDICARE'S BENEFIT-BURDEN BALANCE SHEET

If Medicare had a balance sheet that listed the benefits it provides to older Americans, the list would be long and many grateful seniors would testify to how their life is better because of it.

On the other side of the balance sheet are the liabilities, or burdens, that Medicare enables. This side of the ledger includes the human cost of medically inappropriate tests, surgeries, and treatments; the financial cost borne by Medicare and seniors; lost work time for family members who care for them when they return home from the hospital; the opportunity cost of money wasted that could have added value to someone's life; and the cost to the federal government to borrow money to pay bills that doctors and hospitals submit for medically inappropriate interventions.

Medicare's balance sheet should be all assets and no liabilities. Unfortunately, the liability side of the balance sheet is becoming more populated. Medicare spends too much money that doesn't make life better for seniors and, in fact, makes it worse.

The inappropriate use of medical care and the risk of consequent deprivation of health is no secret in the medical community. More than 40 percent of primary-care doctors say that their patients receive medical care that is unnecessary, according to a survey whose results were published in the *Archives of Internal Medicine*. Many Americans agree. One-third of them say they have had medical care they thought was unnecessary or duplicative.

TAKING MORE FOR THEMSELVES,
LEAVING LESS FOR SENIORS

At the 2008 Republican National Convention, the slogan "Drill, Baby, Drill" was used to express support for domestic oil drilling as a source of domestic energy. A similar slogan, "Bill, Baby, Bill," is the unspoken mantra among many health care providers about unbounded opportunities to bill Medicare.

A consulting industry flourishes that helps hospitals, doctors, and other health care providers maximize the amount of money they bill Medicare and private insurance. Conferences are conducted every year in hotels around the country to show doctors and their staff how to inflate the bills they send to Medicare.

While providers should be paid justly for work they do, Medicare allows enterprising minds to use the system in ways that are good for business but not good for seniors. Medicare is perfectly designed for abuse.

To illustrate, a marketing company website describes how it helps its physician clients "maximize revenue" and "attract new patients." Peppered with testimonials from doctors expressing appreciation for the company's services, the website quotes a satisfied customer, a cardiologist, saying, "My revenue is up 20 percent." The company teaches doctors "exactly what works to bring referrals flooding into your practice even from doctors you don't even know." Its website expresses empathy for embattled cardiologists facing competition from other doctors for business. "It's no secret that more and more general practitioners are now offering diagnostic heart procedures in-house, keeping patients they used to refer to you for themselves," the company says on its website. "And why not? It's just good business."

What is wrong with this picture? A doctor has an ethical obligation to refer a patient to the most qualified doctor. Yet the business of Medicare encourages doctors to keep as many patients as they can for themselves and attract new ones without considering who is most competent to diagnose and treat a person who is ill. Patients become pawns in the Medicare business.

The marketing firm has tips for gynecologists to "attract more of the specific patients you want—infertility cases, for example, and cash-generating cosmetic services that attract more higher-reimbursing patients." These marketing tactics encourage doctors to perform nonessential procedures and discourage them from providing essential preventive care and treatment. The sales pitch sets up a bias against lower-income patients and seniors on Medicare in favor of higher-income, cash-paying patients.

For surgeons who perform bariatric surgery on those who want to lose weight, the company tells doctors, "You know your challenges all too well: Media stories scaring away patients who are considering gastric bypass or lap-band surgery. Or, low-paying HMO or Medicaid cases are starving your practice of revenue. With all these challenges, how will you attract more of the cash-paying, elective bariatric cases you want, that pay you up to 4 times what insurance reimburses? . . . Proven bariatric marketing techniques will show you how to rebalance your caseload with more cash-paying, elective cases and fewer HMO and Medicaid patients; overcome your referrers' and patients' misguided fears about surgery."

By downplaying the very real risks of gastric bypass and lap-band surgery, marketers discourage doctors from telling patients about treatment alternatives and the risks of surgery. By doing so, they promote unethical medical practice. Informed consent is a patient's legal right. Glossing over the risks and treatment options to make a "sale" is unsavory at best.

Marketers urge oncologists to "sell" themselves to attract more patients. Oncology billing teams help doctors "increase average billings and reclaim money" they have been "leaving on the table." Firms claim they can increase billings by as much as 10 to 30 percent.

The only way that oncologists can attract more patients is to scramble among themselves for a limited number of patients and increase how much they bill for each one, which burdens people who are already struggling with a life-threatening disease. An experienced oncology nurse practitioner who worked in a private oncology practice witnessed the burden firsthand.

To increase office revenue, the oncologist began to require his patients to come to the office weekly to obtain lab results rather than tell patients their lab results over the phone. They had to make more trips to the doctor's office that were not medically necessary and pay the copay for each visit. Marketing glitz is not helpful to sick people battling cancer. As doctors, hospitals, and everyone else take more for themselves, seniors pay more when they can least afford it and least feel like it.

"PAY, BABY, PAY"

If you are a boomer, you are following in the footsteps of your parents, who were the program's earliest beneficiaries. They may have lived during the Great Depression and witnessed its deprivations and day-to-day means of survival, whether it was mending socks, switching off lights, saving used wrapping paper and ribbons for the next birthday, and urging children to clean their dinner plates.

Early rumblings of a program to help Americans have access to health care began in those dark days in the 1930s when unemployment skyrocketed and men in ragged suits sold apples and pencils on the street. President Franklin Delano Roosevelt established Social Security and had his sights on health care, too, but that would have to wait.

When the greatest generation breathed a collective sigh of relief at the end of World War II, they came home to build a robust economy. They earned the wealth that helped to make Medicare possible and were deservingly its early beneficiaries. As President Lyndon Johnson said, "We must not neglect, in their age, those who have given a lifetime of service to their country."

Boomers have experienced an unprecedented growth in their standard of living in the past fifty years, made possible by the groundwork laid by their parents. Most boomers enjoy a material standard of living their parents could only imagine. Looking ahead, that standard of living is at risk of eroding because of health care. Out-of-pocket health care spending will increase faster than income, taking an ever-larger bite.

Here is what boomers can expect based on projections from the Urban Institute, a Washington-based organization that conducts research on social and economic issues. If health care costs grow more than in recent decades, nearly two-thirds of older Americans will spend at least 20 percent of their Social Security and other income on health care in 2040. These numbers don't include the cost of a nursing home, home care, and other long-term care, which can wipe out even financially well-off families.

If the White House and Congress require seniors to pay more for Medicare, their disposable income will be cut further. Employers will continue to eliminate retiree health benefits and boomers will pick up that slack too. They will have less money to spend for housing, food, transportation, and other goods and services that provide a good quality of life. Tradeoffs will be nonnegotiable. A home might be an apartment rather than a house. An SUV might be traded in for a smaller vehicle or none at all.

Health care spending has already lowered the standard of living for so many Americans who pay a large share of their income for medical care and forgo other necessities. Bankruptcy has been the only option for those who can't manage to pay for both.

In 1981 only 8 percent of families who filed for bankruptcy did so in the aftermath of a serious medical problem. In 2007 two-thirds of bankruptcies were filed because of medical issues, mostly high medical bills. Most medical debtors were well educated and middle class, and three-quarters of them had health insurance. Many families who filed for bankruptcy had health insurance, but it didn't cover the additional out-of-pocket costs.

Wise use of health care resources is the rising tide that lifts all boats. Unwise use causes the tide to recede and lowers all boats. A window of opportunity exists now to start the tide rising again. By choosing wisely and eliminating inappropriate medical care, boomers and seniors will have a better chance of enjoying the standard of living they deserve.

A Country without Red Lights

$\mathcal{H}$ere is a story of how Medicare helps millions of seniors every year. It is also a story of how Medicare officials try valiantly to manage a half-a-trillion-dollar program without red lights.

If you look at a clock and can see its outline but not the hands that tell the time, you might have a leading cause of blindness called age-related macular degeneration. It can cause permanent loss of central vision, making reading and driving impossible. The condition has earned the label of a new scourge of aging.

A drug named Lucentis made by Genentech, a San Francisco–based firm that is part of the giant Swiss pharmaceutical company Roche, was approved by the Food and Drug Administration (FDA) to treat the more severe form of age-related macular degeneration. The focus of treatment is to stop the progression of the disease. The drug is injected into the eye and works by preventing blood vessels from growing in the center of the retina, called the macula. When vessels leak and bleed, objects look blurry. With treatment, 95 percent of people have their vision stabilized and don't continue losing vision. About one-third regain some vision. Injections are given every month for up to two years.

It took a year from the time the FDA approved the drug to when the drug became available for sale. The most serious form of age-related macular degeneration needs to be treated immediately because there is a narrow window of six to twelve months when treatment is most effective, before blood vessels break and bleed and a scar forms in the back of the eye. When a scar develops, vision cannot be restored. Age-related macular degeneration can take years to develop, but vision loss can occur abruptly, often within a few days or weeks.

Wanting to help their patients avoid blindness, eye doctors began to use Avastin, which is similar to Lucentis and made by the same company. Avastin is injected directly into the eye. It is inexpensive and costs as little as thirty to fifty dollars for a monthly treatment.

Avastin is approved by the FDA for treating certain cancers by preventing blood vessel growth and choking off blood supply to tumors. It is similar to Lucentis but has not been approved by the FDA for treatment of age-related macular degeneration. Eye doctors began to use it off-label, without FDA approval, which is legal, because of the urgency to treat patients as soon as possible.

When Lucentis came on the market, it was priced at two thousand dollars per monthly injection, or about fifty times the cost of Avastin. With the Medicare 20 percent copayment, the drug costs nearly five thousand dollars a year, an impossible expense for many seniors. Genentech did not seek FDA approval for Avastin as a treatment for macular degeneration.

Citing unspecified safety issues, Genentech announced in 2007 that it was limiting the availability of Avastin to treat macular degeneration. The American Academy of Ophthalmology and eye doctors protested the planned change, claiming that the action would hurt lower-income seniors who couldn't afford the higher-cost drug. Skeptics questioned the safety concerns about Avastin, asserting that the company wanted doctors to use only the more expensive Lucentis. Bowing to the pressure, the company backed off and said that Avastin would still be available to doctors.

Avastin is sold in 100 mg or 400 mg vials for use in cancer treatment. Much smaller amounts are needed for treating age-related macular degeneration. Pharmacists repackage the drug in smaller vials in a sterile environment so doctors can use it.

The federal government funded studies to compare the two drugs to learn if they were equally effective. In 2012 the National Institutes of Health reported that Avastin is as effective as Lucentis. After two years of treatment, two-thirds of patients had driving vision (20/40 vision or better), a remarkable improvement.

The median age of people in the study was over eighty years. All adverse events experienced by patients were tracked whether or not they were caused by the treatment. Forty percent of people who had Avastin had a serious adverse event, primarily a hospitalization, and 32 percent of people receiving Lucentis had such an event. It isn't known if the treatment caused the adverse events. Fewer doses were associated with a higher rate of adverse events, which suggests that the drug itself didn't contribute to poor outcomes. The safety of the drugs continues to be monitored.

WHY MEDICARE CAN'T PAY
THE LEAST COST FOR A DRUG

An audit conducted by the Office of Inspector General (OIG) in the Department of Health and Human Services in September 2011 found that if Medicare had paid only for the lower-cost Avastin, Medicare and seniors would have saved about $1.4 billion. Seniors paid nearly $300 million of this amount in higher copayments.

Congress hamstrings Medicare officials by preventing them from paying the least cost for drugs under Medicare Part B. While most drugs are covered under Part D, Medicare Part B pays for a limited number of drugs, such as injections like Avastin and Lucentis that require a physician to administer them.

In 2008, officials in the Bush administration tried to save money by paying the least cost for a drug. In response, the drug manufacturer and a Medicare beneficiary sued the federal government for unlawfully limiting the amount of money it paid. In this case, the patient had a lung condition called chronic obstructive pulmonary disease, or COPD. The plaintiffs claimed that the "least costly alternative" is contrary to congressional intent.

The federal district court in Washington, DC, ruled that Congress specified in legislation how Medicare should pay for drugs. The court noted that Congress went to great lengths to establish payment rates in minutely detailed legislative language. It ruled that Medicare officials cannot pay the least cost on behalf of the public because Congress did not give them the authority to do so.

WHY MEDICARE OVERPAYS FOR DOCTOR VISITS

Here is another example of how Medicare is required by Congress to pay for medical care in the most expensive way possible. If a senior goes to a doctor's office for a fifteen-minute office visit, Medicare will reimburse the doctor. The patient will pay a 20 percent copayment. If the doctor sells his or her practice to a local hospital, the next time the senior goes to see the doctor, Medicare will pay 80 percent more for the same fifteen-minute office visit. The care is the same, but Medicare pays almost double. Seniors pay more money out of pocket too.

The extra payment is a "facility fee," presumably to offset higher overhead costs. It encourages hospitals to buy doctors' practices so they are a part of a hospital's network. Consequently, more office visits are taking place in hospital-owned facilities. The extra cost drives up Medicare Part B premiums and copayments.

The nonpartisan Medicare Payment Advisory Commission advises Congress on Medicare policy and recommended that Congress permit Medicare officials to pay doctors the same amount wherever the service is provided. The powerful hospital lobby will fight hard to allow its members to keep charging Medicare as much as they can, as often as they can.

WHY MEDICARE PAYS TOO MUCH FOR MEDICARE ADVANTAGE PLANS

Twelve million Medicare beneficiaries are enrolled in Part C of Medicare, called Medicare Advantage. More than half of them are in plans offered by a handful of large companies including UnitedHealthcare, Humana, Kaiser Permanente, and Blue Cross and Blue Shield.

Medicare has been paying the plans more than the amount it would pay if seniors opted to stay in the traditional Medicare program. President Obama's health care reform law has a provision to reduce payments to the plans so they are more consistent with traditional Medicare program costs.

While health care reform pared back payments, the Obama administration created a loophole to give more money back to the plans through a revised bonus scheme. Health plans are rated for the quality of care they provide to seniors. Under Medicare law, only plans with four stars out of a maximum of five can receive a bonus. Medicare officials extended bonus payments to plans that had only three stars or more, which diluted the intent to reward only the highest performers. According to the Medicare Payment Advisory Commission, Medicare paid an additional $2.8 billion in 2012 for bonuses to average performers, a policy that is difficult to justify on the basis of quality and cost.

The nonpartisan Government Accountability Office (GAO) recommended that the bonus program be cancelled. Pegged at a total cost of $8.3 billion over several years, the program is unlikely to improve quality because most of the money is going to plans that are average, according to the GAO. In a letter to Secretary of Health and Human Services Kathleen Sebelius, the GAO's general counsel, Lynn Gibson, questioned Medicare's legal authority to implement the more generous bonus program. The health insurance industry will persist in trying to block any reduction in payment.

That Medicare pays more than it should reveals how the health care industry has acquired an entitlement mindset. It believes it is entitled to keep getting more of Medicare's money irrespective of merit, propriety, or other compelling public interests for how the public's money should be spent.

MEDICARE'S CHIEF DESIGN FLAW

For Medicare to become a reality in 1965, President Johnson made concessions to hospitals, doctors, and insurance companies. They would not negotiate prices with the government. Instead, they wanted to determine how much Medicare should pay them. The then-nascent industry included hospitals and doctors who had become accustomed to billing the dominant private health insurer at the time, nonprofit Blue Cross and Blue Shield, at prices they deemed appropriate.

Medicare contracted with Blue Cross and Blue Shield plans to process the bills from hospitals and doctors. The plans claimed that implementation of Medicare would have been impossible without them. Representatives of hospitals and doctors, among others, were on the boards of directors of Blue Cross and Blue Shield. In this way, they governed the companies that processed the claims they sent to Medicare for payment.

Johnson capitulated to the industry players because they had the upper hand and he needed them to participate. Otherwise, Medicare could never be implemented. It was agreed that Medicare would pay doctors the "usual and customary" rate rather than a negotiated price. By doing so, a nascent industry became the price setter, and the government and seniors became the price takers. The imbalance of power sent a message to would-be entrepreneurs that Medicare was open for business.

Medicare law set the stage for an open-ended entitlement program without enough red lights. No limit was placed on the amount of money that seniors and taxpayers would pay in perpetuity. This is exactly what the special interests wanted, and that is exactly what America got. This is why Medicare spending each year is equivalent to Sweden's gross domestic product and growing with no end in sight.

The United States departed from health care policies in Europe and Canada that installed red lights to limit the excesses of private industry. Here at home, the industry disparages the "socialist" systems in other countries. The complaints are a masquerade for chafing about rightful limits that governments impose on companies' ability to make excessive amounts of money at the expense of the financial solvency of governments and their citizens.

Once Medicare gave the health care industry a green light, the floodgates opened. Lobbyists insert language in legislation detailing how much the government will pay them. In the courts, industry lawyers challenge every step Medicare takes that might limit company profit. They file frivolous lawsuits against anyone who stands in their way, sapping the time, energy, and resources of opponents. Public policy is made by bulldozing their way around Washington.

The health care industry's control over the direction of Medicare policy has reached beyond the tipping point. Medicare officials lack the authority to rein in the industry. They are relegated to managing a program without authority from Congress to install red lights or make sure that existing ones operate. Any system without red lights is headed for a crash. When the crash occurs, people will be hurt. That is when people will wake up and wonder why the red lights weren't working.

Americans woke up in 2008 when the banks caused a crash that nearly pushed the country over the financial cliff. It happened because the financial industry controlled the levers of power in Washington, systematically weakened regulatory agencies meant to enforce common-sense rules, and blocked any action to hold them accountable.

In March 2012 the U.S. House of Representatives voted 223 to 181 to repeal the Independent Payment Advisory Board, the fifteen-member panel authorized in the health care reform law slated to keep Medicare from spiraling out of control. Once again, Congress stopped the installation of a red light at a busy intersection. The Senate did not take up the bill. If it had, President Obama threatened to veto the legislation.

BRACE FOR THE CRASH

Countries don't work when they don't have red lights. Both Republicans and Democrats have removed Medicare's red lights. What will the crash be like? Here are two scenarios.

Scenario #1

The government is falling further behind in paying doctors and hospitals that provide services. It has a backlog of unpaid bills that already stands at $1.9 billion and is on track to grow so large that doctors, hospitals, and pharmacies may cut off services because the government can't pay them. If nothing changes, in five years the government will have twenty-one billion dollars in health care bills it can't pay. In the meantime, health care spending is being slashed.

Scenario #2

A medical equipment supplier received an order from a local hospital for a heart-monitoring machine. The supplier decided not to fill the order. It is awaiting payments from hospitals that haven't paid their bills. That's because the government doesn't have enough money to pay hospitals the money it owes them. The owner of the medical equipment company stopped paying regular salaries to his eight employees and cut their hours.

The first scenario is unfolding in Illinois and was reported in the spring and summer of 2012 in the state news media. The second scenario took place in Greece and was reported in the *Financial Times* in the summer of 2012 during the Eurozone turmoil.

The U.S. economy is far larger than that of Greece and can paper over small crashes relative to the size of the economy. In both countries, though, people and governments have lived beyond their means. More productive countries are willing to lend them money. Greece has reached the point where lenders are reluctant to loan them more money. The United States is on the same path, and the impact of the austerity measures that are inevitable will be far reaching domestically and internationally. Brace for the crash.

Part III

HOW WALL STREET DETERMINES THE CARE YOU GET

Medicare has morphed from its original intent as an entitlement to help seniors avoid impoverishment because of medical expenses. Today, it is an entitlement for American businesses, made possible by a persistently powerful nexus between Wall Street and Washington. This nexus will determine Medicare's future if a countervailing force fails to dilute its influence. Its impact is visible today. In part III we examine the point of impact of Wall Street on seniors as it trickles down into their daily lives in ways as basic as getting out of bed in the morning.

Chapter 8 gives a glimpse of where the smallest part of Medicare—the 1 percent spent on hospice care—actually goes. It is a window on the sea change that has taken place in the overall Medicare program in the past three decades. It reveals how hospice care evolved from its early days as a voluntary mission of caring for people when they reached life's end. With Medicare funding, nonprofit hospices were established around the country to care for seniors and their families. Today, half of all hospices are for-profit. The chapter is a front-row seat on how private equity firms buy and sell hospices and use dying seniors as instruments of private gain.

In towns all across America, the Wall Street–Washington connection plays out in imperceptible ways. Chapter 9 makes the connection real. Bangor, Maine, was a battleground state between nonprofit dialysis treatment clinics and a for-profit multinational company that wanted to buy them. The proposed sale triggered scrutiny by smart local residents who wanted to know more about the multibillion-dollar company that wanted to come to town to take care of some of the sickest and most vulnerable members of their community. This chapter traces their discovery about what it means when Wall Street comes knocking on the door of Main Street. Behind the suits and PowerPoint presentations is a reality that only the most determined and curious skeptics will piece together.

The ties that bind Wall Street and Washington are long and storied. Chapter 10 tells how politics and business have been intertwined since the country's birth. Today, the ties are drawing tighter than ever as Medicare is on track to consume a growing share of the federal government's budget. With the prospects of even more Medicare largess looming, Wall Street occupies Washington to ensure the money is ferried its way. The relationship plays out in debates on Capitol Hill. The battle over federal regulation of medical devices that millions of seniors use to keep their joints moving and hearts ticking is a perfect case study. During the debate, the people most affected were relegated to spectator status, sidelined as decisions were made behind closed doors. The debate provides a sneak preview of who will make decisions that determine Medicare's future.

· 8 ·

Medicare's One Percent

$\mathcal{M}$itt Romney's 2012 presidential campaign brought private equity firms out of the closet. A cofounder of Bain Capital, a Boston-headquartered private investment firm, Romney was a flashpoint for a debate about private equity. His personal fortune was pegged at up to $270 million, most of it from his years working at the firm. During a campaign that was all about the economy and employment, the source of Romney's wealth stirred a vigorous debate about whether private equity kills jobs or creates them.

Private equity can help companies that might otherwise go belly-up regain their footing. Upstate New York flatware maker Oneida, whose knives, forks, and spoons decorated dining-room tables in homes across America, had been battered by low-cost production in China and was on the verge of collapse until private equity investors swooped in to try to rescue it under friendly terms.

Private equity firms are better known for their notorious dealings, scooping up thriving companies, loading them up with massive amounts of debt, stripping them of their money, and flipping them to new owners while walking away with outsized profits. While raiders reap multimillion-dollar gains, the workers reap a harvest of pink slips.

The most infamous private equity deal is the twenty-five-billion-dollar buyout of RJR Nabisco in 1988, the subject of the movie *Barbarians at the Gate*. The transaction epitomized the pinstriped corporate raiders battling each other to take control of a company with no regard for the employees making the Oreos.

Private equity investors have cropped up in unlikely places. They have been buying hospices that were established to care for the terminally ill and turned what was once a mission into a racket. Although hospice care accounts for just 1 percent of all the money Medicare spends each year, it is a microcosm of the sea changes that have occurred in Medicare in the past thirty years.

WHEN PRIVATE EQUITY INVESTS IN BUSINESSES FOR THE TERMINALLY ILL

Sprinkled around rural Kansas are twenty branch offices of for-profit Hospice Care of Kansas, based in Wichita. It has local offices in Anthony, Kansas, a small town with about three thousand people, and Great Bend, with fifteen thousand residents and named for its location on the big bend of the Arkansas River.

Hospice Care of Kansas was one of several hospices owned by a Texas company, Voyager. In 2004 Voyager was bought by a thirty-five-billion-dollar private equity firm, Apax Partners, whose investments include a buffet restaurant chain in China, a clothing store in Europe, and an automotive internet marketing company in New England.

Hospice Care of Kansas and Voyager catapulted into the crosshairs of federal investigators over allegations of fraud brought to light by a seasoned nurse, Beverly Landis, who was dismayed by what she observed when she came to work at the hospice. The hospice had a laserlike focus on increasing enrollment. Medicare pays hospices about $150 a day for each person regardless of the services provided. The more people they enroll, the more they get paid.

To receive hospice care, two doctors, including the hospice medical director, certify that a person is terminally ill and is expected to live six months or less if the disease that is draining life away runs its normal course. He or she agrees to forgo Medicare coverage for curative treatment but can leave hospice care at any time and go back to the regular Medicare program to receive full benefits. Hospices provide benefits not usually covered by traditional Medicare such as social-work services, pastoral care, and bereavement counseling for family members after their loved one passes away.

Thankfully, a limited number of people are terminally ill. So how do hospice employees keep enrollment climbing in small towns and cities in Kansas?

Employees at each branch office were given enticing incentives to boost enrollment. According to court documents, the company sponsored enrollment campaigns in which employees were promised an all-expense-paid trip to Cancun, Mexico, if they maintained enrollment above 725 patients for thirty consecutive days. The "Summer Sizzle," "Christmas Cash Blitz," and "Fall Frenzy" were the names of other promotions the hospice sponsored to keep the pressure on their employees to enroll more people, according to the federal investigation. Staff were threatened with termination or a reduction in hours if the number of people enrolled in the hospice dropped below targets.

The hospice billed Medicare for providing services to people who were not dying, a clear violation of Medicare rules. Outside consultants hired by the hospice warned the company that it was at risk of billing Medicare for people who were not eligible. Up to one-third of the patients in one of the hospice service areas were not dying.

The hospices hired marketing and sales staff who used tactics similar to those of drug company sales people, who buy lunches for doctors and their office staff, according to a *Bloomberg* investigation. True to form, hospice employees brought menus from a local steakhouse to doctors' offices, where the staff selected the entrees and desserts. Hospice employees delivered the food. In return, the hospices expected doctors to refer patients. Referrals were richly rewarded with retreats to luxury destinations and free family vacations at a local lodge. Nursing homes provided a ready supply of patients, so the hospices paid nursing home doctors handsomely, up to four thousand dollars a month for working about a day a week, *Bloomberg* reported.

Once people were enrolled, managers required employees to keep them enrolled as long as possible, even when they were feeling better and no longer needed hospice care. Nurses were coached how to write in medical records that patients were sicker than they actually were so the hospice could continue getting paid. Federal court documents revealed that they were instructed to avoid words and phrases that might suggest a patient was improving, a signal that the person is not appropriate for hospice. Training documents instructed staff to "remember to chart negative" and not use phrases such as "stable" or "may possibly not be appropriate for hospice."

A nurse wrote in an e-mail that a patient's condition was likely chronic, not terminal, that the patient had gained weight, and that the patient's oxygen saturation was okay. Despite this assessment, the nurse wrote in the patient's medical record that the patient had declining function and should continue services.

When doctors and nurses determined that a patient was no longer eligible for Medicare's hospice benefit, the company stalled and established a thirty-day discharge process. After that period ended, the company imposed yet another eligibility review. The company president and vice president ignored the recommendations of doctors and nurses and weighed in on whether a patient should continue in hospice, all the while forgoing curative treatment.

E-mails from a vice president on consecutive days to the branch executive directors stated, "Let's please try to minimize these [live discharges]," and "We really have to find a way to stop all these live discharges." In other words, the hospice needed the revenue from each patient to meet financial targets.

The hospice kept a lid on spending. Voyager's regional vice president chimed in and sent an e-mail to several hospice offices telling them they needed to tell their staff to stop the "constant requests for resources." The e-mail stated, "It is time that we help [staff] understand. . . . To remain financially viable, we must stay within our budgets. Of course, with that said, 'high water covers a lot of stumps.' In other words, when we get our census up, that will free resources."

The hospice wasn't starved for cash. It made a lot of money for its private equity investor, Apax, which sold Hospice Care of Kansas and Voyager in 2010 for eighty million dollars, four times its original investment, *Bloomberg* reported. The federal investigation into allegations of fraud was underway the same year and apparently wasn't a deal breaker.

The buyer was Harden Health Care, which used loans and equity from Kohlberg Kravis Roberts (KKR), the same private equity firm that claimed victory in the buyout of RJR Nabisco. KKR owns a minority share of Harden. The president of Harden Health Care is a former president of Bank of America in Austin, Texas.

The same year that Apax sold the hospices, a record seventeen hospices were bought and sold. Prices for hospices have risen significantly. Private equity firms buy hospices with the intention of holding them five to seven years, maxing out Medicare reimbursement, and selling them for a profit. Investors and top management typically have little, if any, background in health care.

In June 2012 Hospice Care of Kansas and its parent company, Voyager, agreed to pay $6.1 million to resolve allegations that they billed Medicare for seniors who were not terminally ill. The government accused the companies of enrolling seniors and keeping them enrolled when they were not dying, instructing employees to write misleading information in medical records, and linking nurses' compensation to enrollment targets.

WHEN THOUGHT BECOMES REALITY

Why do companies become like this? Every system is designed to achieve the results it gets. Hospices that operate under laws governing for-profit corporations are required by those laws to maximize investor profits. Boards of directors of corporations have a fiduciary duty to fulfill this purpose and can be sued by shareholders if they fail to do so.

The mandate rolls downhill to executives, who are held personally accountable for meeting financial targets. Managers and employees, who enroll patients and interact with them, know that their livelihoods depend on making the numbers.

The wisdom of the sages says that what we think, we become. If the thoughts of hospice company executives or private equity firm partners are to make money, they will permeate the entire enterprise from top to bottom.

Thoughts become words. Emails from company executives translate the mandate of making money into words. The words become the talk of morning staff meetings, employee performance reviews, and bonus time. They are infused into the conversations between doctors and patients and their grieving sons and daughters.

Words become actions. Doctors, nurses, and social workers tell grandmothers and grandfathers they are going to die, forcing them to confront their mortality when, in fact, they are not dying. Collateral damage doesn't appear on the radar of company higher-ups. The radar is turned off. Tasks are performed, disconnected from the sacred moments when life is indeed coming to a close, and the corporate office could care less. All that matters is the single-minded goal of keeping revenue up, expenses down.

Actions become habits. Company events whip up a frenzy of excitement about the prospect of putting another person in a hospice bed whether he or she is dying or not. Actions become habits reinforced by a reward system peppered with money and recognition. Punishment is unceremoniously meted out when money, status, or a job is lost for failing to pledge unwavering fealty to corruption of human purpose.

Habits become norms. The norms create expectations for the people who come to work every day. Informal, unspoken rules govern expectations and behaviors. Attitudes toward the sick are formed and reinforced. They determine whether the sick are perceived as human beings worthy of the compassion Mother Teresa would render, or just another cog to meet monthly enrollment targets and be greeted with feigned concern and caring. Norms define the character of a place, the people, the collective, the corporation.

Norms create a parallel universe. Companies absorbed in their pursuit of the bottom line create their own world with its own contrived reality. It enables the words that tell a daughter that her father's life is coming to an end when it is not.

The cause is won; a job is well done. Competition replaced cooperation. Tension usurped harmony. Targets snuffed out emotion. Moneymaking supplanted caretaking. Success is celebrated over drinks at happy hour.

The nurse at Hospice Care of Kansas bore witness to company norms that were out of sync with the honorable norms society intended. When management blew her off for failing to march in lockstep with the contrived reality it created, she blew the whistle and federal investigators enforced society's norms of what is right and just.

A person who seeks medical care doesn't know the thoughts, actions, habits, and norms of the hospital, clinic, or doctor's office into which he or she steps. On the surface, the offices may look alike, with the usual chairs stacked side by side in the waiting room, magazines on the table, and staff seated behind desks. But the hidden culture is what matters. An outsider will have a tough time grasping it.

A hospital or hospice may have a patient's bill of rights or its latest inspection certificate dutifully posted on a wall. What matters is the unspoken thought that shapes everything that everyone does. The company you keep really does matter. Is there loyalty and devotion to you, the patient? In the end, that's what counts. But who is counting and what are they counting?

Loyalty is not counted, nor is compassion. Money is counted. Large hospices owned by publicly traded companies generate profit margins nine times higher than those of large nonprofits and three times higher than privately owned for-profit hospices of similar size. It doesn't matter that investor-owned hospices, whether private equity or publicly traded companies, skimp on care to patients. Thought becomes reality.

The money may bring short-term glee, a new multimillion-dollar house for an investor, or simply another paycheck for a top manager. Deep and abiding satisfaction will never be found in such remuneration. It can have an opposite, corrosive effect, for it was borne of human-induced suffering.

Nurses, social workers, and others who work in places whose character is compromised by slavish fidelity to investors may feel divided, even pained, at the constraints placed on them. As a condition of their employment, they must render to their Caesar what is expected, all the while seeking in their hearts to care for an elderly woman or man as if she or he were their own mother or father, but cannot. Divided lives are lived. Employment options in small towns are limited. Minds are fraught with worry and hearts quietly break while going through the motions, wishing it were different, desiring to live divided no more.

A nurse who works in a hospital on the East Coast told the story of a patient she had cared for whose life was coming to an end. Management objected to her spending too much time with him, but she did so anyway as her colleagues "covered" for her by caring for her other patients.

When expressions of human compassion are discouraged in the name of efficiency and metrics, humanity is suppressed. Dehumanization strips away the qualities that make us in the image of something much greater than ourselves.

WHEN HOSPICES DON'T NEED
PRIVATE EQUITY BUT GET IT ANYWAY

Private equity is typically used to bring working capital to a company to help it expand, or bring new products to market, or restructure the company's operations, management, or ownership. Does private equity bring any value to hospice care?

Hospices don't need large infusions of capital for physical infrastructure because most people are cared for at home. Highly labor intensive, the biggest constraint to hospice expansion is finding enough qualified nurses to care for patients. Private equity funding isn't needed to invest in innovation since hospice care has an established approach. Nor is any highly specialized management required.

While private equity investments can offer value to investors, its value to patients is not so clear. Investors flip hospices similar to how real estate speculators flipped houses during the mortgage boom. Speculative investment didn't help the housing market or homeowners. Flipping hospices doesn't help patients. They are mere commodities to attain market value.

FROM PLUMBERS TO HOSPICES

The number of new federal investigations of alleged hospice fraud jumped 50 percent from 2008 to 2010, according to the U.S. Department of Health and Human Services. In 2010 more than thirty cases were opened following whistleblower suits brought by former hospice employees and others who alleged hospices defrauded Medicare. Here are recent cases that illustrate how endemic fraud has become in the care of the dying.

- The largest for-profit hospice in the country, Vitas Healthcare, is under federal investigation for Medicare fraud. A former manager of the company filed a whistleblower lawsuit in federal court in November 2011, accusing the hospice chain of enrolling people who were not terminally ill. Vitas is owned by the same company that owns Roto-Rooter plumbing.
- In January 2012 the U.S. Department of Justice joined a whistleblower lawsuit against AseraCare, an Arkansas-based hospice that operates in nineteen states, alleging that the company enrolled people who were not terminally ill and kept them there as long as it could. According to a Kaiser News Report, hospice employees went door-to-door in public housing projects to find people they could label as terminally ill and enroll them and rode along with Meals on Wheels volunteers to find prospective customers.

- In 2009 a Birmingham, Alabama, for-profit hospice company, SouthernCare, entered into a $24.7 million settlement with the federal government over allegations that it enrolled people in hospice care who were declared terminally ill but were not.
- In 2006 national for-profit hospice chain Odyssey Healthcare paid $12.9 million to settle allegations that it submitted false claims to Medicare. The Dallas-based company allegedly enrolled people who were not terminally ill.

THE MISSION

Hospice care didn't start out this way. It began as a charity with the noblest intentions of nurses and doctors to alleviate suffering. The transformation from mission to business to racket didn't take long, a mere twenty years.

Saratoga, New York, is the home of the National Women's Hall of Fame. One of its honorees is Florence Wald, the former dean of the Yale University School of Nursing, who was recognized for her pioneering work to bring hospice care from England to the United States.

A native New Yorker and graduate of Mount Holyoke College, her mission started in the 1960s to provide comfort to people whose life was coming to a close. She and her like-minded colleagues knew that people were being treated for diseases such as cancer even when doctors knew it was futile.

Dr. Wald invited Dr. Cicely Saunders from London to talk about her work to alleviate suffering. Saunders had been a nurse during World War II and witnessed immense suffering. She became a doctor and devoted her life to relieving suffering. For her visit to New Haven, she brought photographs of patients nearing the end of their lives before and after they had been treated for their pain and other distressing symptoms. The difference was remarkable. That is the difference Florence Wald wanted to make.

She stepped down as dean of the nursing school and traveled to London to learn how Dr. Saunders cared for patients and brightened their lives. She studied the hospice's organization and management. Wald returned to Connecticut and began to provide hospice care in the United States. Wald and her like-minded clinical pioneers made themselves available to people whenever they were needed, whether in a hospital, at home, or in a nursing home. This approach was radical because the care followed the patient. Usually, the patient has to fit into the system. Hospice was meant to be about the people it served.

In the beginning, doctors, nurses, and social workers were volunteers. Communities established hospices with charitable donations. Hospice care sought to alleviate suffering from the excruciating pain of a metastasizing cancer and the shortness of breath that can feel like suffocation.

Wald and other pioneers testified on Capitol Hill to encourage members of Congress to include hospice as a Medicare benefit. Beginning in 1983, with money from Medicare to pay for hospice care, Wald's vision of relief of suffering could be realized.

In the early days, hospice organizations were established as non-profits with a duty to their communities. The designation was not merely a tax status for purposes of the Internal Revenue Service. The organizations were nonprofit in spirit as well as the letter of the law. The aim was to provide a community service. They had only one master, and that was the people they served. As hospices became for-profit, they suddenly had two masters, investors and the sick.

FROM MISSION TO BUSINESS TO RACKET

Wald and her colleagues established the first hospice in the United States, the Connecticut Hospice in Branford. Disagreements surfaced shortly after the hospice opened. Years later in an interview, Wald talked about these disagreements. Her democratic style of management clashed with that of a businessman from the Wharton School of Business at the University of Pennsylvania who had a top-down decision-making style. "He needed to be the boss," Wald said.

"While I was on vacation, he had given the Board of Directors an ultimatum: either he was to come on as the CEO and I was to leave, or he would leave. So, they first asked me to resign and I refused to do that, so I was forced out. . . . In hindsight, it seems like the wrong thing. . . . The Wharton Business School won out." The takeover was a harbinger of what was to come.

Fledgling voluntary hospices needed to evolve to become formal organizations if they were to be prepared to care for hundreds, if not thousands, of people each year. New institutions had to be established and their financial soundness assured, which required skills different from those needed to care for people at the bedside. Both are needed to fulfill the mission.

Many hospices have tried to keep the mission alive. No mission, no margin is the mantra. In fact, without their mission fully intact, they won't be able to get it right. Many dedicated people work in for-profit hospices too, but the fiduciary duty of their governing boards is to shareholders, not patients.

At a visit to a place that cares for the terminally ill that has stayed true to its mission, we were told of a young man with a tumor on his neck the size of a soccer ball. Nurses had gently wrapped his head and neck with a white cloth to minimize his family's distress when they came to see him. They provided the young man a measure of dignity in his final days. There were no staff vacancies at this place, and staff turnover was zero. They had a singular commitment to the patient. No enrollment targets were set, no incentive programs were established to recruit patients who were not terminally ill. Their purposeful mission was evident the moment we walked in the door and the doctor who greeted us said, "The only restraints we use in this hospital to keep our patients safe are the arms in which we hold them."

FROM JEEPS TO HOSPITALS

The transformation in hospice mirrors the changes in hospitals, home health care, and nursing homes that bill Medicare.

If you live in Boston and need to go to the hospital, one of them may be owned by private equity firm Cerberus Capital, which bought six Catholic hospitals that the Archdiocese of Boston sold in a fire sale. This is the same Cerberus Capital that bought Chrysler, the maker of the Jeep, in 2007, an acquisition that went south.

If you live in Detroit, the Blackstone Group controls Vanguard Health Systems, which bought the Detroit Medical Care System.

If you need nursing home care, the Carlyle Group is one of multiple private equity firms that bought 1,876 nursing homes from 1998 to 2008, according to the Government Accountability Office.

If you need home health care, the four largest publicly traded home health care companies were investigated by the U.S. Senate Finance Committee for billing for unnecessary services. Three of them, Amedisys, LHC group, and Gentiva, were found to have manipulated Medicare by encouraging employees to boost the number of home-care visits when patients didn't need them.

Corporate executives at Gentiva drove their fifty-one management teams to compete with each other to gain more profitability. Whether people needed the services didn't appear to be a top priority. Administrators assigned team names to each region of operation, such as the Mid-Atlantic Spider Monkeys and the Carolina Killer Bees.

The Senate committee report said that, at best, the practices are abuses of the Medicare home health program and at worst, they may be examples of for-profit companies defrauding the Medicare home health program at taxpayer expense. The companies maintain they have done nothing wrong.

The story has a similar plot to that of JPMorgan Chase, which tried to make up for lost profit after the economy tanked in 2008 by creating its own mutual funds and marketing them to unsophisticated mom-and-pop investors to turn a profit. JPMorgan brokers said they felt pressured to recommend to customers the company's products even when less-expensive and better-performing investment options existed, the *New York Times* reported. Rather than being financial advisors, they were pressured to make the sale even if the customer was given a bad deal.

Brokers who give investment advice are not required by securities laws to have a fiduciary duty to act in the best interests of their clients. But doctors and nurses have a duty to act in the best interests of their patients, a duty conferred by their medical and nursing licenses. Yet as a condition of their employment, many are expected to be salespersons to increase the organization's margin, whether it is a hospice, a home-care agency, or a hospital.

Trust is the essence of health care. The purpose is to help people in the most intimate of ways in the most compelling times of their lives. Boards of directors and senior executives need to be stewards not only of the public's money but of the lives entrusted to them. Without trust, health care becomes nothing more than a financial transaction in which a person produces their body, things are done to it whether needed or not, and money is collected.

WHAT IT MEANS FOR YOU

Who pays for the millions of dollars in the billable hours of law firms to defend against indefensible claims of Medicare fraud? Who pays for the money frittered away on the phalanx of highly paid investment advisors, lawyers, and accountants hired every time a hospice, home-care agency, nursing home, or hospital is bought and sold?

You do. If you are working, the money comes from the Medicare payroll taxes deducted from your paycheck. Your money is used to pay the cost of Medicare Part A, which includes hospital, skilled nursing, hospice, and home care. These providers use a portion of your money to cover the cost of transactions that are extraneous to care of the sick. It is funneled to the care and feeding of investors. This is not part of the deal Americans think they are getting. Yet you are paying for it.

Seniors and boomers facing retirement have a good chance of spending their final days in a hospice where the humanistic dimension has waned. Nearly half of the people who are on Medicare use hospice care at some point, and the percentage is growing. Meanwhile, for-profit hospices have multiplied and account for about half of all hospices. They are crowding out nonprofits, which are on the decline.

The generation of mission-oriented leaders who established hospices as a community service around the country have moved on, leaving a vacuum in public-spirited leadership at the helm of a vital part of America's health care continuum.

Good people will do the right thing and provide humane and compassionate care no matter where they are. Boomers will need to seek and find them. They may work outside the mainstream, forging a path on their own, because the rough currents of twenty-first-century health care in America whisk nonconformists to the sidelines. It is the only place where they can survive and thrive, doing the work as it was meant to be done, in deep devotion and service to humanity.

· 9 ·

When Wall Street Health
Care Comes to Main Street

$\mathcal{O}$n a spring morning in Bangor, Maine, forty-two-year veteran nurse Kathy Day read an article in the *Bangor Daily News* about a nearby hospital that was planning to sell three of its clinics where people with kidney failure are treated. Eastern Maine Medical Center had signed an agreement to sell them to a Fortune 500 company, Colorado-based DaVita, one of the largest for-profit dialysis companies in the country.

At first glance, the sale might appear promising for the community. *Forbes* magazine rated DaVita that year as one of the most admired companies. The company is innovative, according to *Forbes*, and it caught the eye of stock-picker guru Warren Buffet, who owned 6 percent of the company's shares.

Kathy wondered aloud, "Why would EMMC sell out fine, locally run and controlled dialysis clinics to a Fortune 500 corporation from out of state?" She was determined to find out. Along the way, she learned what happens when Wall Street health care comes knocking on the door of Main Street.

OWNERSHIP MAKES A DIFFERENCE

Medicare began to pay for treatment for kidney failure in 1972 to anyone regardless of age. Kidney failure is a death sentence within three weeks of onset. Common causes are poorly managed diabetes, high blood pressure, and kidney disease.

Treatment is called dialysis and is provided in centers usually three times a week for three hours. It mimics the function of real kidneys. Blood is allowed to flow a few ounces at a time through a special filter that removes wastes and extra fluids. The blood is then returned to the body.

Before Medicare began paying for dialysis treatment, community leaders held fundraisers to build and operate dialysis treatment facilities. Not everyone who needed treatment could receive it. After Medicare started to pay, for-profit companies began to dominate the business.

Eastern Maine Medical Center's clinics have been among a diminishing breed of nonprofits in a world of for-profit dialysis treatment. Two large companies, DaVita and Fresenius, own 60 percent of all dialysis centers in the country. Another 20 percent are owned by smaller for-profit firms.

Does ownership matter? Proponents of corporate health care say they can deliver high-quality care more efficiently than nonprofits. Opponents say that the primary duty of companies is to their stockholders, not patients. When a company has to balance profits and people, the temptation is too great to put profits before people.

A HOT STOCK

From an investor's point of view, there is a lot to like in dialysis treatment. Medicare is a stable and rewarding revenue source. As rates of obesity and diabetes soar, the number of people dependent on dialysis will increase. From the vantage point of for-profit companies, it is a lucrative opportunity. From a public health perspective, the trend is exceedingly worrisome.

A month after the proposed sale in Bangor, the company revealed a pending $4.4 billion deal to buy a large operator of medical groups and physician networks around the country so the company could expand to provide more than dialysis treatment. The company's stock was billed as "hot" by investment analysts.

Nurse and advocate Kathy Day believed that the dialysis clinics owned by the hospital in her community provided good care. "Information about bad care often trickles down to me because I am a patient safety activist and advocate," she said. "I have never heard anyone complain about their treatment." Kathy believes that the hospital has been keeping its promise to the community, saying, "It has stayed true to the charitable donors who donated money to pay for a four-year-old facility on the west side of Bangor."

Kathy and her family have experienced substandard care firsthand. Four years earlier, her eighty-three-year-old father, John McCleary, broke his leg and went to a local hospital. He succumbed to an infection that he likely acquired when he first went to the hospital. The infection was triggered by bacteria that are resistant to antibiotics. Since then, Kathy has become a nationally recognized advocate to encourage hospitals to work to prevent hospital-acquired infections. People on dialysis treatment are susceptible to infections. She became interested in the sale of the dialysis clinics because she wants to ensure that people in her community receive good care.

NOT-SO-HOT CARE

Researchers who studied the differences between for-profit and non-profit dialysis facilities and published their results in the *New England Journal of Medicine* found that for-profit ownership was associated with higher mortality and a lower chance of being placed on a waiting list for a kidney transplant. The authors pointed out that for-profit treatment facilities might be reluctant to refer patients to be evaluated for transplantation because they lose revenue if patients receive a new kidney and no longer need dialysis.

What caused the higher mortality rates? People with kidney disease lose the ability to make red blood cells and become anemic. They are given drugs that stimulate the body to produce more of them. Medicare paid for the drugs based on the amount that was administered. If patients received higher doses, the dialysis centers received more money. For-profit dialysis centers used a lot more of the drug than their nonprofit counterparts.

The company that manufactures the anemia drug, Epogen, is Amgen, based in Thousand Oaks, California. It was selling the drug to dialysis company chains at volume discounts that encouraged them to use more of it. DaVita's contract with Amgen included volume discounts and other stipulations. If the dialysis company could not meet them, its earnings would be adversely affected. The contract provision was a powerful motivator for dialysis centers to use as much of the drug as possible. According to one of DaVita's annual reports, the drug accounted for about a quarter of its total revenue from its dialysis services.

For many years, Amgen insisted that people on dialysis who took the drug would be healthier because more was better. Drugs to treat anemia racked up the single largest Medicare drug expense. Amgen did not achieve this blockbuster distinction based solely on the alleged benefits of the drug. It enlisted a powerful member of Congress to be its spokesperson. As the *Washington Post* reported in an extensive review of the rise and fall of the drug, "Congress forced the regulators to let the drugs flow." Its actions harmed untold numbers of unsuspecting Americans who thought more medicine would help them. They had been duped.

Leading the charge in the Senate on behalf of the company was then-senator Arlen Specter from Pennsylvania, who wanted Medicare to pay for higher doses of Epogen. At the time, Specter controlled the purse strings at the Medicare agency. Amgen had enlisted the right person in Washington to advocate on behalf of its drug.

Specter grilled the top Medicare administrator in the late 1990s, Nancy-Ann DeParle, wanting to know why government bureaucrats decided that Medicare would not pay for drug dosages that exceeded FDA recommendations. Here is an excerpt from the exchange on Capitol Hill from the *Washington Post* that captures the essence of the Wall Street–Washington link and how it hurts people on Main Street:

> "Ms. DeParle, what is your level of expertise in this field? What is your background and training?" Specter asked. "I am a lawyer, sir," she replied, according to a transcript. "So there is no special level of expertise that you have to make this kind of an evaluation?" Specter, a lawyer, wanted to know. Medical experts on her staff believed that Epogen was being overused, she said.

Physicians working for Medicare who tried to put patients' interests first didn't stand a chance against Senator Specter and the lobbying onslaught behind the scenes. Forced to scrap their plan to limit the amount of the drug that Medicare would pay for, they agreed to pay for a higher dosage that Senator Specter wanted. Amgen stocks jumped 6 percent the day Medicare announced it was increasing the amount of the drug it would pay for. Amgen made it to the Fortune 500 list, thanks in part to Washington insiders who unlocked government coffers.

U.S. senators don't always know what they are talking about. Numerous studies found a link between larger doses of drugs to treat anemia and higher mortality. The groundbreaking research confirmed that people who received higher doses had an increased risk of heart attack, stroke, and death.

More than a decade after the hearings hosted by Senator Specter, the FDA issued a stern warning in 2011 saying that drugs used to treat anemia in patients with chronic kidney disease were dangerous to the heart and doctors should avoid using them or greatly reduce the dose they give to patients.

The following year, DaVita settled a whistleblower lawsuit and paid fifty-five million dollars for allegations of drug overuse. A former employee of drug maker Amgen accused DaVita of administering more of the drug than was medically necessary to boost profits. The company was also accused of double billing Medicare for the drug that was left over in vials and reused. DaVita denied any wrongdoing. The company's practices in the use of anemia drugs are under investigation in other states, and a federal grand jury is investigating the company's financial arrangements with doctors.

If the public is to have confidence in companies that perform a service that makes a difference between life and death, they need to trust them. Actions such as these give the public plenty of reason to question their trustworthiness.

The United States has among the worst outcomes for people on dialysis compared to other countries, according to the conclusions of a Boston meeting of physicians concerned about the poor care that people on dialysis receive. More than 20 percent of people treated for kidney disease die each year. More than 70 percent die after five years. Mortality can be as high as 40 percent in the first year of dialysis treatment. Fewer than 20 percent are able to go back to work. Improving outcomes has been nearly impossible. It is hard enough to make improvement in the practice of medicine. It is even harder when corporate interests seek to maintain the financial status quo.

Dialysis treatment is Medicare's for-profit child, born and raised with Medicare's silver spoon. Medicare has enabled bad habits at the behest of Congress, who sets the rules that Medicare officials are required to carry out. The offspring is an adult that lives off an entitlement thanks to a generous public that trusts more than it should.

The collateral damage is invisible, borne by nameless, faceless people and their families all across America. No one is held to account. Top executives are given a free pass. If companies are given the responsibility to care for the sick but instead deceive and harm them, Medicare should take its business elsewhere. Many doctors, nurses, and others of high character are willing and competent to provide compassionate care for fellow Americans, who deserve at least that much, and more.

TRUST IS EARNED NOT BOUGHT

Most people on dialysis don't know about the high-level corruption that has taken place in the dialysis business. They are too busy struggling with their illness and treatment. They have to trust the people who take care of them because they have precious little energy to advocate for themselves.

Kathy Day wanted to know how patients are treated at dialysis facilities so she could understand the character of the company that wanted to set up business in her community. She talked with people from around the country who have been outspoken about their treatment and concerns with substandard care.

She learned that patients have been dismissed from dialysis centers for rightfully raising questions and concerns about the quality and safety of their care. When they are dismissed, people become desperate because they will die without treatment. If dialysis patients in rural Maine were dismissed for pointing out safety concerns, their only option would be to drive many hours each way three times a week to be treated at a different dialysis center, an impossible situation for many of them. They are captive to their illness and the place where they receive treatment. That's why Kathy believes it is important to know whether a local dialysis provider is trustworthy.

These concerns are not new. During hearings in Congress in the 1980s, dialysis patients testified about being threatened, coerced, intimidated, and finally denied their life-sustaining treatment. Little has changed in thirty years. That's because accountability for providing substandard care is weak or nonexistent.

WHAT HAPPENS IN BANGOR DOESN'T STAY IN BANGOR

Kathy Day wondered why the hospital wanted to sell its three dialysis clinics. Was it because the economics of providing dialysis services has changed?

Medicare had been paying dialysis centers a set rate for treatment plus a separate amount for drugs, laboratory tests, or other services. Under this payment approach, dialysis centers had the incentive to overuse drugs, which benefitted companies such as Amgen as well as DaVita. Medicare abandoned this method and now uses a bundled payment. Treatment centers are given a set dollar amount for each patient. Within that amount they have to provide all services to patients, including drugs and lab tests.

Here is a possible scenario that could have triggered the proposed sale. In fall 2011 Amgen negotiated exclusive deals to supply its drug to DaVita and Fresenius, which together own 60 percent of the dialysis treatment centers in the United States. Contracts with both companies include discounts and rebates. Did Amgen offer to sell its drug to Eastern Maine Medical Center at a price that was too high for the hospital to afford under the new bundled payment system because it didn't have the market clout of the big chains? The public will never know the reason that the hospital wanted to sell its dialysis clinics.

The new payment system is open to its own set of abuses. Arlene Mullin, a former dialysis technician who testified before Congress years ago about abuses in treatment centers, offers insight on what will happen. She witnessed firsthand the changes that occurred when her employer, a nonprofit dialysis treatment center, was sold to a for-profit company intent on saving money.

Staff received minimal training. Many technicians had only a high school degree and received about six to eight weeks of training. "It was like having two years of college crammed into six weeks," she says. "The staff didn't even know they might be killing patients because they weren't trained." Companies save money by using more lower-paid technicians and fewer nurses.

"Within the first week, I had to take care of four patients at once, rather than three," she says. "I didn't have time to take blood pressures within the first half-hour that the patients were on dialysis because I was too busy getting other people set up for their treatment."

The company used its own labs to test patients' blood because it was cheaper. But it took longer for the test results to come back. "We couldn't identify problems quickly and intervene, and this put patients at risk," Arlene says.

With new incentives for dialysis treatment, the care that people receive will change. As dialysis treatment goes, so goes Medicare. Boomers and seniors are at risk for experiencing less personalized care, more assembly-line-type treatment, more staff with lower levels of training, higher risk of mistakes, treatment decisions based on profitability not medical necessity, and lack of interest to improve the care provided to patients.

QUESTIONS TO ASK WHEN MULTINATIONAL COMPANIES COME TO YOUR COMMUNITY

When for-profit corporate health care comes knocking on the door in your community, it is important to ask what kind of company it is and what is its purpose. A quick Google search can reveal media stories and other information about the company and its character. As a corporation, its intention is to make money for its investors. It is legally obligated to its shareholders. Here are questions to ask yourself, your neighbors, and leaders in your community:

Where Does the Money Go?

When health care facilities are locally owned, Medicare reimburses them for the cost of providing care to people in their communities and the money will go to that community. With large chains of dialysis centers, hospices, or home-care agencies, a portion of the money received from Medicare leaves the community and goes to corporate headquarters to pay company stockholders and the salaries of company executives, who are working to build more business. Should the money that comes from Medicare stay in the community?

Who Is in Charge?

Nonprofit facilities are required by law to have a governing board whose responsibility is to ensure that the institution serves the community and is accountable to it. When a for-profit company takes ownership of clinics and hospitals, its fiduciary responsibility is to the people who own the company, not the community. There is no local board to hold the company accountable. Communities lose control of health care facilities when they are sold. Corporate executives answer to headquarters, not to communities.

Who Is Accountable?

If the people in your community have concerns about substandard care, who is accountable and where does the buck stop? Does it stop with a manager in a regional office of a multinational company? If so, the employee is accountable to his or her supervisor, not to a local community or nonprofit board that is required by law to represent the public's interest. Not all nonprofits uphold their duty to the public, however. But at least a legal obligation exists that can be enforced.

Do Doctors Have Divided Loyalties?

Health care companies have a variety of compensation schemes for doctors. Doctors may own stock in the company or the company may lease clinic facilities from doctors, who in turn make money from rental income. Their loyalty is divided between the interest of the patient and that of the company. This can happen in nonprofit organizations too. People who are sick don't want doctors with divided loyalties.

· *10* ·

Wall Street and the Federal Government: Born Forty-Eight Seconds Apart

*W*all Street is best known as the epicenter of the country's financial system. It occupies another prominent place in American life.

George Washington was inaugurated the first president of the United States on Wall Street. The ceremony took place on the balcony of Federal Hall in 1789, whose address is what is now 26 Wall Street.

The first United States Congress convened in Federal Hall. It served as the first U.S. Capitol. The Bill of Rights was born there, right on Wall Street.

Three years later on May 17, 1792, twenty-four stockbrokers gathered outside 68 Wall Street under a buttonwood tree to sign an agreement that would establish the rules for buying and selling bonds and shares of companies. The signers of the so-called Buttonwood Agreement were the pioneers of what became the New York Stock Exchange, whose address is 11 Wall Street, a forty-eight-second walk from Federal Hall, according to Google maps.

The business and political elite literally grew up across the street from each other. It should not be surprising that the ties that bound them at birth have remained strong throughout the generations. Today, the nation's political hub is a brief seventy-two-minute plane ride from the country's financial nerve center.

In a classic symbiotic relationship, the president and members of congress need Wall Street to provide the capital investment to generate jobs and economic growth. When the economy fails, their political fortunes fail too.

In turn, Wall Street needs elected officials to protect their profits from taxes and keep regulatory scrutiny at bay. They want access to the public's money to grow their businesses. The dependence on public money is woven through the balance sheets of American companies, as the health care firms on the Fortune 500 list can attest.

Mutual need and benefit transcend political parties. Both Democrats and Republicans are friends of Wall Street. The friendship is lucrative for all. For his reelection bid, President Obama presided at a $35,800-a-plate fund-raising dinner on the Upper East Side of New York with deep-pocketed bankers, private equity firms, and hedge fund managers. A few months earlier, the wife of Jon Corzine, former governor of New Jersey and former chief executive of Goldman Sachs, held a fund-raiser for Obama at her home. Her husband later came into the spotlight as CEO of MF Global, which lost nearly two billion dollars in hard-earned money from people who trusted the system to work for them.

Not to be outdone, Mitt Romney was guest of honor at a $50,000-a-plate dinner at the Southampton home of billionaire business-man David Koch, who steered millions to the Romney campaign and Republican congressional contests. Mitt Romney's presidential cam-paign netted more of Wall Street's money than the Obama campaign.

What's at stake for Wall Street? The federal government spends a lot of money every year—$3.7 trillion in 2012. With that much money in play, Wall Street wants as much as it can get. Little wonder that the Acela trains and the Delta and U.S. Airways shuttles between Washing-ton and New York are always busy.

ACCESS WASHINGTON

Steven Baker from Bloomington, Minnesota, is an Air Force veteran and father of two children who learned firsthand who has access in Washington and who doesn't. As a twenty-seven-year millwright, he helped build the Metrodome in Minneapolis and Camp Snoopy at the Mall of America. He traveled to Washington to meet with his member of Congress to talk to him about a medical device that was implanted in his elbow after he was injured at work. The device failed just four months after the surgery. When he moves his elbow, it makes a popping or creaking sound. To repair the damage, Steven had another surgery, but it was unsuccessful and the gnarling pain is unabated.

Steven wanted to let his congressman, Eric Paulsen, a Republican who represents Bloomington, know how important it is for Congress to ensure that medical devices are safe before they are sold and implanted in peoples' bodies.

Steven was given an appointment with a young staff member in Congressman Paulsen's office in Washington, and he traveled from Minnesota to the Cannon House Office Building on Independence Avenue across from the Capitol. During Steven's meeting with the young staffer, Congressman Paulsen popped in the room, waved to Steven, and left. He didn't shake hands with a constituent from his district who had traveled nearly three thousand miles round-trip to give him an important message that he hoped would improve public policy and benefit Americans around the country. Paulsen took substantial amounts of money from the medical device industry to loosen, rather than strengthen, device safety.

"Your voice gets muted before you are even done with the meeting," Steven says. "From my experience, ordinary people just get smothered up. Nothing ever gets done. It's lip service without ears. I don't walk in with a basketful of money for them. But corporations do because government is for sale."

OCCUPY WASHINGTON

A few blocks from the White House, the Occupy Wall Street movement protestors pitched their tents in the fall of 2011 and winter of 2012. The temporary tents in McPherson Square and Freedom Plaza were a statement about Americans who felt disenfranchised in their own country. While the aims of the protests were diffuse, the movement diagnosed an ailing America, a predicament deeply felt by many Democrats and Republicans alike. A country that was formed to be a government of the people, by the people, isn't that way anymore. A small cabal has amassed undue influence on government and society to the detriment of both.

As the tents of the Occupy Wall Street movement were taken down, a very different and permanent movement keeps its stakes firmly in the ground. This is the Occupy Washington movement. The occupiers don't sleep in tents. Rather, they wear Burberry and Brooks Brothers suits and live in lavish condos overlooking the U.S. Capitol and in big houses in the Virginia and Maryland suburbs with manicured lawns and Brinks security systems.

This permanent occupation is a reason that Washington and its suburbs are relatively immune from economic downturns. During the Great Recession, unemployment rates were lower than in other parts of the country. The usual explanation is the large federal government workforce and federal contractors who live and work there. The $3.5 billion annual lobbying business is the other explanation.

The money trickles down to the coffers of Tysons Galleria, the high-end shopping mall in the northern Virginia suburbs that was once farmland along the Potomac River. On any night of the week, restaurants and bars in Washington; Bethesda, Maryland; and Clarendon in Arlington, Virginia, are teeming with customers. The Great Recession was a mild blip. New restaurants open and are jammed on weekends and weeknights. These places don't look like most others in America where the ravages of persistent unemployment reign.

A bumper sticker on a car parked in a tony Clarendon neighborhood of North Arlington reads, "Invest in America: Buy a Congressman." In the same trendy micro real-estate market, cocooned from the reality of housing misery in the rest of the country, six brand-new $1.5 million houses were built in a year and sold in a flash.

A closer look reveals cracks in the veneer. A Harvard Law School graduate is a barista in a coffee shop in downtown DC. A graduate of the London School of Economics is unemployed and trying to make ends meet by making flower arrangements for churches. As places of worship cut back their spending even in high-income communities, his business is shrinking. He spends his days in Barnes & Noble reading books and magazines.

The Occupy Washington machine continues to operate at full throttle. Lobbyists need staff to draft legislation to give to members of Congress to insert in congressional bills. They need legions of people to write issue briefs to make their case. They hire watchdogs who watch every move in Congress and the executive branch. They need watchdogs to watch the other watchdogs. Opposition researchers dig up negative information on opponents.

Communications and public relations firms make millions of dollars from lucrative contracts to test and create messages for the Washington elite. Trade associations buy full-page ads to sway an influential readership. The Washington Metro is plastered with ads targeted at staffers on Capitol Hill, in the White House, and in government departments and agencies.

No longer does the *Washington Post* have a monopoly on political news in the capital city. With *Politico*, *Roll Call*, and *The Hill* circulating on Capitol Hill and K Street, political news is a big money maker. The politics of issues—who says what and who disagrees with whom—is the headline grabber. Substance takes a back seat.

THE MAD SCRAMBLE

When it comes to Medicare, the mad scramble in Washington is about getting a piece of the growing share of the country's gross domestic product that will be spent on the thirty-three million additional people who will be covered by Medicare by 2030.

How much money is up for grabs? In 2011 the total value of goods and services produced in the United States was about fifteen trillion dollars. One percent of that amount is $150 billion a year. Medicare already spends nearly 4 percent of the country's income, or close to $600 billion, with more to come.

The money will be divided among hospitals, drugs companies, doctors, home health care, hospice, dialysis treatment centers, durable medical equipment providers, and everyone else that relies on Medicare to make money. While it is hard to know how the spoils of politics will be divided, one thing is certain. The health care lobbying machine will be humming in high gear for years to come. The industry will pay to play, having spent half a billion dollars in 2011 to lobby, a small down payment on billions in future gains.

Where does the money come from to pay the bar tabs and restaurant checks for elaborate dinners? It comes from a slice of the Medicare pie paid by the 156 million Americans who dutifully pay their Medicare payroll taxes, millions who pay federal income taxes, and the millions of Medicare beneficiaries who pay premiums and copayments.

For a preview of how the mad scramble over Medicare will play out, hints of the script can be found during the skirmishes on Capitol Hill in fall 2011 when more than four hundred companies, unions, trade associations, and other groups lobbied the Joint Select Committee on Deficit Reduction, the debt supercommittee. According to the Center for

Responsive Politics, the health care industry showered the most money on members of the supercommittee. Drug companies and hospitals were the most generous.

The hospital industry paid for television ads urging seniors to call their members of Congress and tell them not to cut Medicare payments to hospitals. The cuts would threaten the health of seniors, the ads said. They featured seniors who were indignant that Congress would dare touch hospitals. The industry gave the impression that it was looking out for seniors. Nothing could be further from the truth.

Behind the scenes, the hospital industry pressured Congress to push the financial burden of hundreds of billions of dollars in debt reduction on older Americans rather than trim wasteful spending in their institutions and tighten their belts. The American Hospital Association (AHA) organized hundreds of hospital leaders to trek to Capitol Hill and urge their elected members to increase the eligibility age for Medicare from sixty-five to sixty-seven and increase the premiums that seniors pay for visits to doctors.

Bernie Sanders, a senator from Vermont, wrote a letter to the president of the hospital association, Richard Umbdenstock, saying he found it "disgraceful" that the association was actively working to postpone older Americans' eligibility for Medicare. "With close to 50 million Americans currently uninsured and millions more underinsured, it is indefensible that the AHA would promote changes in Medicare that would not only increase the number of uninsured seniors but would also make care more expensive for those still covered under the program," Sanders wrote.

Gridlock in Congress staved off any supercommittee action. Seniors had a reprieve, but the political playbook is a sign of times to come. The strategy of the health care industry bears similarities to how Goldman Sachs put its interests before the interests of its clients. As pressure mounts to control Medicare spending, the health care industry will advance its interests at the expense of grandmothers and grandfathers, mothers and fathers, boomers and seniors all across America.

BOOMERS AND SENIORS VS. THE MEDICAL DEVICE INDUSTRY

Terry is a sixty-six-year-old retired boat builder who moved to Florida. Five years ago he was told he had an irregular heartbeat. His doctor said he could die instantly from cardiac arrest and recommended that a pacemaker and defibrillator be implanted in his chest. The pacemaker would keep his heart beating regularly, and the defibrillator would deliver a small electric shock to restore normal rhythm if his heartbeats became irregular. Electrodes, or thin wires, connect the defibrillator directly to the heart. Since then, Terry remembers only one instance when he felt a low-level shock in his chest.

Not long after the procedure, he received bad news. The defibrillator wires, called leads, that weave through his heart could fracture and fail, giving unnecessary shocks or none at all. Terry asked his doctor if the faulty wires could be taken out and replaced. His doctor said it would be more risky to replace them than to keep them intact. He was one of about 170,000 Americans affected by the faulty wires.

Every month, Terry goes to the doctor to have the wires tested. The test does not offer any assurance that the device or the wire leads are working properly. He worries that the defective wires could fail at any time. "When the wire leads fail, you croak," he said bluntly in a Long Island accent.

Terry is especially irked that the FDA allowed the device to be sold. "In June 2007, the FDA knew the wires were suspect, but they didn't take action," he says. "I had the procedure in October 2007. This is the reason I'm aggravated. The FDA should have acted sooner."

More than 250,000 people worldwide were adversely affected by the type of defibrillator that Terry had implanted, according to Dr. Gregory Curfman, an editor at the *New England Journal of Medicine* who testified at a congressional hearing. The defibrillator is called the Sprint Fidelis and was manufactured by Medtronic. With inadequate premarket testing and a fast-track FDA approval process, corners were cut, resulting in a "devastating" situation for patients, Curfman said.

To understand Terry's dilemma, imagine you own a car and receive a letter in the mail from the manufacturer, perhaps General Motors or Toyota. The letter says that the brakes are defective and there is a small chance they won't work when you press your foot on the brake pedal. The defect cannot be fixed and you can't exchange the car for a new one. You have no choice but to drive it for the rest of your life knowing there is a small but real chance the brakes could fail. The longer you have the car, the more the risk increases. Imagine, too, that the National Highway Traffic Safety Administration, which oversees vehicle safety, knew that the brakes were faulty. You bought the car when the government knew they were defective but failed to act in time.

WHY SAFETY MATTERS

Mesmerized into believing that science is on the verge of creating a bionic human whose parts can be replaced when they wear out, Americans are easily led to believe that if a product is innovative it must be better than other products already on the market. Television advertising beams into Americans' living rooms and spreads the hype that replacing a hip or knee with a new and better one is a cinch, like buying a new set of tires for a car.

Machines are never perfect, and neither are the people who design and make them. That is why the safety and effectiveness of new medical products need to be tested before they are sold and placed in the inner sanctum of a human body. Innovation is essential to the country's economy, but it is only beneficial if it does good and not harm. Testing doesn't stifle innovation. It enables innovation that the world envies.

Katherine Korgaokar knows firsthand that medical devices labeled as innovative are not always better. She told a congressional committee about an artificial hip joint she had implanted. The surgeon said the new design was better than other artificial joints and should last twenty years or more. It was made by DePuy, a division of the New Brunswick, New Jersey, company Johnson & Johnson, best known for making Band-Aids and baby powder.

Pain free after the surgery, Katherine could do all the activities she loved to do. Four years later, she received a letter from her surgeon saying that the manufacturer recalled the hip joint because of excessive wear and tear on the metal parts that caused pieces of metal debris to be released into her body. A blood test revealed she had excessive levels of toxic cobalt and chromium that were used to make the joint. The metal particles can damage the bone and tissue surrounding the joint and harm the heart, nervous system, and thyroid gland.

Katherine had surgery to remove the joint and replace it with another one, a procedure that is not for the faint of heart. The pain during recovery is much worse than after the first operation, and mobility is more impaired. Successive operations affect the muscles, tendons, and bones in the hip, making it less stable. The joint is more prone to become dislocated, an excruciating experience.

In testimony before the U.S. Senate, she said she had thought that medical devices are extensively tested in the human body before being sold. Then the wake-up call came. "I had no idea that devices could be 'fast tracked' by the FDA with little or no testing," she told Congress.

The FDA can approve a new device if it is similar to an existing one without requiring testing in humans for safety and effectiveness. The vast majority of medical devices such as replacement hips and knees are in this category. In fact, the FDA can approve a new device that is similar to an existing one even if it was defective and removed from the market.

An overwhelming majority of Americans want tighter rules to ensure that devices are safe and effective before they are sold, according to a *Consumer Reports* poll. Ninety-one percent of people who responded said implants should be safety tested before being sold, even when similar implants are on the market. Sixty-eight percent of those respondents felt strongly about it, saying they "definitely should" be safety tested.

The stakes are high. Seventeen percent of people surveyed said they have a medical implant, and 47 percent have a family member or close personal friend who has one. These numbers are bound to increase as boomers realize their hearts, knees, and hips are not the same as when they were teenagers.

WHY IS THE UNITED STATES IN THE DARK?

Katherine's experience with metal-on-metal implants was not isolated. Nearly one hundred thousand people had the same type of joint implanted. The FDA received over five thousand complaints about the metal-on-metal hips. Dr. Curfman of the *New England Journal of Medicine* referred to the harm as a "public health nightmare."

Fortunately, doctors in Australia and the United Kingdom were tracking which hip joints worked best. They kept a log, or registry, of patients in their countries who had hip replacement surgery. Information was collected about the type of artificial joint used, the manufacturer, and how well each patient fared. Doctors noticed patterns in the data on tens of thousands of surgeries. Not a single new artificial hip or knee introduced in the five years they studied lasted longer than older models that cost less money. One of the newer designs for hip joint replacement that didn't perform well was the metal-on-metal model used in Katherine's first surgery. In fact, it was more likely to fail much sooner than expected.

Why did Australian and UK doctors have information about the joints but U.S. doctors did not? Manufacturers don't want them to collect comparative information about the safety and effectiveness of their products and report the results to the public. Sales will plummet if their products fare poorly in the competition. At best, companies are not confident about the quality of their products. If they were confident, they wouldn't hesitate to put their product up against any competitors' product. At worst, companies know their devices are subpar and can't stand up to scrutiny.

Even with this public health "nightmare," the medical device industry lobbied Congress to speed up the FDA approval process and roll back safety standards. In a highly contentious debate, the Republican majority on the House Oversight and Investigations Committee held hearings that criticized the FDA for delaying approval of devices and putting the brakes on innovation and job growth.

Pressure came from wealthy venture capitalists who invest in small start-up companies. They want a quick green light from the FDA to speed the return on their investment. A big manufacturer with deep pockets might buy a small venture capital–backed firm to bring a newly approved device to market. Investors reap handsome returns quickly before the product is sold and any defects surface.

Congressman Paulsen from Minnesota, home to device maker Medtronic and other device firms, sponsored a bill that would have made it easier for devices to move through the approval process quickly without human testing and monitoring for safety defects. Mr. Paulsen's campaign received $74,000 from device companies and their industry backers, according to the *New York Times*.

Democrats on the congressional committee—Henry Waxman, Frank Pallone, Diana DeGette, and John Dingell—were irked by the lack of balanced content in the hearings and wrote a letter to their Republican counterparts, Fred Upton, Joseph Pitts, and Cliff Stearns, urging them to have testimony on the potential dangers to patients if medical devices are not appropriately regulated.

Democrats revealed that brain stents are another device approved by the FDA without human testing. Designed to open up a blocked artery in the brain after a stroke to prevent another stroke, they were approved by the FDA using the fast-track process. A study funded by the National Institutes of Health examined 451 people who had a stent implanted in an artery in their brains and found that 15 percent of them had a stroke or died within thirty days. Those who were treated with medication did better, and far fewer, 6 percent, had a stroke or died.

NOT THE BEST WAY TO CREATE JOBS

Congressman Adam Kinzinger, a Republican from Illinois, claimed that industry-favored legislation will ensure an FDA review process that will "eliminate the threat of sending jobs overseas." A closer look at the jobs argument from the vantage point of the person on the gurney waiting to go into the operating room for a replacement knee or hip gives new meaning to job creation.

Assume that ten thousand of the nearly one hundred thousand people who had defective metal-on-metal hip implants had a second hip surgery to remove a defective joint and replace it with a safer, more reliable model. Defects create a lot of work for doctors. If an orthopedic surgeon performs two hip replacements a day for twenty days each month, twenty surgeons will be fully employed for a year. Nurses in the operating rooms, recovery rooms, and surgery floors are employed.

Drug companies will employ people to keep producing the pain drugs that people will need to manage their physical suffering.

Johnson & Johnson and other supply companies will sell more sheets, bandages, sutures, and other materials used during the surgery and hospital stays. Hospitals will have an additional ten thousand patients admitted to their facilities.

Device companies will churn out ten thousand replacement joints. They might be made in the United States, although companies such as device maker Medtronic are hiring people in China for the company's new research facilities. CEO Omar Ishrak said in an interview, "The cost today of engineering talent . . . is much lower for almost as good output." Six months earlier, Medtronic announced it was hiring one thousand skilled workers in China in the next five years. Around the same time, 268 company workers in the Twin Cities were laid off.

Lawyers for patients and device makers will be employed for years handling rightful demands from patients for compensation. People will be employed to take the jobs of those who need repeat surgery and cannot go back to work right away, if ever.

This type of job creation mimics the job creation during the sub-prime mortgage meltdown. Banks approved mortgages for people who did not have the financial means to repay the loan. Yet the mortgage boom created jobs in construction, real estate, and banking until the whole scheme came crashing down. Innocent bystanders were collateral damage. It was not a way to run a banking system. Neither is it a way to run a health care system.

Just as the banks privatized their gains and socialized their losses, nearly bringing the country to its knees, the device industry and its financial backers privatize their gains and socialize their losses by spreading them among people like Steven, Terry, and Katherine who bear the human and financial cost.

The industry, Congress, and the Obama administration ignored the recommendations of doctors and researchers convened by the Institute of Medicine at the National Academy of Sciences who examined the medical device regulatory process. After an exhaustive review, they concluded that fast-track device approval is inconsistent with public safety and should be replaced with a more robust approach. They urged the FDA to cease fast-track approval for a device if it is similar to an existing one that has been removed from the market because of safety defects. Even this commonsense provision was not included in the bill passed by Congress in June 2012 and signed by President Obama.

The legislation excluded reasonable steps to require studies to track the safety of devices once they are sold. Remarkably, if the FDA issues an order for a study when safety concerns arise after a device has been approved, it doesn't have the authority to rescind its approval of the device if the manufacturer fails to comply with the order or if the study shows that the device is unsafe or ineffective.

Boomers and seniors should have access to information on the comparative performance of devices so they can make informed choices. Transparency would motivate manufacturers to create and sell the best and safest products.

The law gave the FDA more than six billion dollars in industry user fees over five years to offset the cost of the device-approval process. *Politico* touted the relative civility that characterized passage of the bill. The medical device industry, the FDA, and legislators on both sides of the aisle agreed early on they would make a deal. Wall Street got what it wanted. That is why legislation sailed through Congress without the usual fireworks in an otherwise deeply partisan legislative body.

In a classic case of regulatory capture, consumers and patients were sidelined. While most don't have technical knowledge of devices and the industry, they have crucial information about product performance that technical experts don't have. They were not welcomed in the policy dialogue. The voices of ordinary citizens, for whom government is supposed to work, were ignored.

Investors' expectations of quick financial returns on complex devices and implants used in the human body are out of sync with the gravity of the intended purpose. It is not easy to produce a new and better artificial knee or hip every few years that can replicate the miracle machine that human beings are born with.

Yet the device industry's business model requires a constant flow of so-called innovative products, hoping a few of them stick. Under pressure from wealthy investors, companies must deliver financial returns. Investors who try to game the stock market want to apply the same rules to game the human body. That's a game no one will ever win. Nature doesn't bow to Wall Street.

The time-frame for healing the body is different from the time-frame that short-term investors seek to reap quick money. Quick returns are incompatible with the long-term investment needed to figure out how the body works and find solutions to ailments that have affected humankind since the dawn of civilization and before that. It isn't like designing a new athletic shoe every season.

In a high-functioning market economy, manufacturers would welcome information about defects in their products so they could correct them and produce a better product that competes with others on the market. There is no well-functioning market in medical devices. Coupled with a dysfunctional regulatory system that fails to protect the public, product defects will continue to proliferate, and tens of thousands of Americans like Steven, Terry, and Katherine will be harmed.

LESSONS FOR SENIORS, BOOMERS, AND MEDICARE'S FUTURE

The medical device debate in Congress reveals how the nexus between Wall Street and Washington affects the lives of seniors and boomers in profound and intimate ways. On the one hand, investors provide the financing needed to design and manufacture products that enable people to live a better, happier life. On the other hand, the same company that makes a life-saving product can sell a product that cripples tens of thousands of people.

The medical device industry's win in Congress and the White House came on the heels of an earlier win in the courts. The U.S. Supreme Court limited the right of people harmed by defective medical devices to seek redress in state courts, according to the ruling in *Riegel v. Medtronic* in 2008. People harmed by defective devices cannot sue in state courts the manufacturers of certain medical devices approved through the FDA's more stringent process, the ruling said. The court reasoned that because the device was approved by the federal government, that approval preempts state laws. Manufacturers are held harmless and do not have to pay for the harm caused by their products.

Since the Supreme Court ruling, lawsuits against medical device manufacturers have been thrown out of state courts. Medicare and seniors pay the cost of harm from defective devices, repeat operations, and doctor visits. It is a classic example of privatized gain by the companies and socialized losses paid by society.

What should boomers and seniors do? Think about questions you would ask when buying a car. How often does the device break down? The doctor should tell you the answer. If the doctor says that the information doesn't exist because the product is too new, it may still be experimental. Find out if there are long-term studies on the model that will be used in your operation. Search online for information about the device in the mainstream media.

If you have hip or knee joint replacement surgery when you are in your fifties, you may need replacement surgery when you are older and the body is less likely to rebound as quickly as after the first surgery. The results probably won't be as good as the first time because your body will have scar tissue and inflammation, which makes a joint less stable.

Find out from the website Dollars for Docs (dollarsfordocs.org) if your doctor is taking money from the company that manufactures the implants. Drug and device company payments to doctors are listed.

The lessons from the medical device industry's win in Congress and the White House may be a harbinger of what is to come for Medicare. Public-interest advocates watched as the industry took command of the legislative process. The advocates were no match for the well-heeled, powerful constituency that, in the end, stopped the government from acting in the best interest of the public.

At the entrance to the New York Stock Exchange on Wall Street is a pediment entitled, "Integrity Protecting the Works of Man." It depicts the robed figure of Integrity as she stretches her arms outward, a symbol of honesty and sincerity.

Seventy-two minutes away at the Lincoln Memorial is the inscription with the noble words from Abraham Lincoln's Gettysburg address, ". . . that government of the people, by the people, for the people, shall not perish from the earth."

May it be so.

Part IV

THE ENTITLED AND THE ENTITLERS: TAKING A SLICE OF THE AMERICAN PIE

An entitlement program is a two-way street. It has givers and takers. In chapter 11 we take a look at the takers, the businesses that lobby for excessive Medicare spending. Takers develop a habit of taking. Habits are hard to break. The first step to break a habit is to name it and acknowledge it. We name the seven habits of an entitlement-based health care industry: it wastes money, tolerates poor performance, resists scrutiny, has reputational immunity, breeds corruption, silences critics, and seeks protection from political elites. Each of these habits affects the health and well-being of seniors and all Americans.

Chapter 12 traces the newest beneficiary of Medicare's entitlement, Wall Street hedge funds. As health care has become populated with more for-profit players than ever, Wall Street investors see opportunity to take a bigger slice of the American pie. We trace how New York–based Marwood Company, whose president is Ted Kennedy Jr., son of the late Senator Edward Kennedy, used connections in Washington to offer hedge fund managers access to high-level Medicare officials who decide the devices and drugs Medicare will pay for.

Not to be outdone, members of Congress have also benefited financially from their proximity to the legislative process. During the Medicare prescription drug debate, Democrat John Kerry made millions buying and selling drug company stocks while he served on the Senate committee that had oversight of the legislation. The chapter ends with a discussion of the STOCK Act, a law enacted in 2012 to deter Washington insiders from trading on inside information.

Chapter 13 takes a deep dive into the world of givers and takers during the 2012 presidential election. We shine a light on the candidates' positions on Medicare and their relationships with the health care industry. Over the years, many of the candidates benefited financially from their privileged connections. Some of them sounded the alarm about Medicare's financial predicament during the presidential campaign yet have added to the program's precarious financial situation by giving more of the peoples' money to the industry.

• *11* •

Seven Habits of an Entitled Health Care Industry

$\mathcal{M}$edicare is known as an entitlement program for seniors over age sixty-five. It is also the largest and most lucrative entitlement-based program for the health care industry.

In 2011 the federal government redistributed nearly six hundred billion dollars from seniors and other taxpayers to hospitals, doctors, home care agencies, skilled nursing facilities, drug companies, device manufacturers, and other providers of services. Millions of seniors benefit every day, and their lives are better because of it. Nonetheless, a substantial portion of the money is wasted on excessive spending that does not help seniors and might cause more harm than good.

Republican congressman Paul Ryan from Wisconsin criticizes Medicare for creating a culture of dependence and entitlement among the public on government-run programs. Today, a senior on Medicare can expect to receive, on average, about $180,000 in Medicare benefits during his or her retirement years. This amount is lost in the decimal points of the billions in excessive, wasteful spending by the health care industry, which has an entitlement mindset and is dependent on Medicare.

An entitlement-based industry does the following:

- Wastes money
- Tolerates poor performance
- Resists scrutiny
- Has reputational immunity
- Breeds corruption
- Silences critics
- Seeks protection from political elites

WASTES MONEY

The amount of waste in Medicare is equivalent to the entire economy of New Zealand. Here is how we came to this startling conclusion. The Institute of Medicine of the National Academy of Sciences estimates that about 30 percent of health care spending does not add value to peoples' health and is wasted. Thirty percent of Medicare's $560 billion in spending in 2011 is about $170 billion. New Zealand's economy produced $162 billion in goods and services that year.

Here is a small example of how the health care industry wastes money. A Midwest surgeon told us the story of a meeting he attended in Washington where Dr. Donald Berwick, former administrator of the Medicare program, was giving a presentation. Dr. Berwick urged the doctors in the audience to be good stewards of health care resources.

The surgeon was motivated by Dr. Berwick's missive. When he returned home, he asked the chief financial officer at his hospital to find out the cost of the supplies in his operating room. The surgeon acknowledged that he never knew how much they cost. Together, the surgeon and the financial officer reviewed the inventory. The operating room had $700,000 worth of supplies. Ten percent, or $70,000 worth, had expired and had to be thrown away. The surgeon whittled down the essentials to $295,000. He could buy less expensive sutures, for example, saving $35,000 a year without any difference in outcomes for his patients.

Spurred by the realization of four hundred thousand dollars in wasted expenditure and the potential for the entire health system to save money, the surgeon met with the CEO of the health system where he worked and challenged him to reap similar savings in all operating rooms. Doing so could save hundreds of millions of dollars in several years by prudently purchasing and managing the inventory of operating room supplies.

The surgeon continued his quest and learned that other well-known teaching hospitals lack inventory control for operating room supplies and waste millions of dollars a year. The absence of the most rudimentary controls suggests that hospitals' other processes are riddled with waste. Businesses in other sectors of the U.S. economy would be unable to survive with such profligate practices.

After months of effort, the conscientious surgeon was unable to convince his hospital to be a prudent purchaser of supplies and equipment. The reason, he said, was "corruption."

Public revelations of health care waste are relatively rare. In contrast, the public learns when the Pentagon pays eight hundred dollars for toilet seats, as it did in the 1980s, and more recently, seventeen thousand dollars for helicopter drip pans that sell for a fraction of the cost. Unlike expensive toilet seats, overly expensive sutures, medical supplies, and equipment are rarely scrutinized in the media because they are shrouded in seemingly specialized knowledge known only to health care professionals.

Many hospital employees can attest to the magnitude of waste in hospitals. A colleague of ours at a teaching hospital told us how his hospital decided to save thousands of dollars a year simply by purchasing a commonly used product from a different supplier. A doctor at the hospital complained because the company that charged a higher price gives him fifty thousand dollars a year for his research. The hospital continued to purchase the more expensive product.

Here is a telling example of an entitlement mindset that encourages wasteful spending and bad medical care. Doctors at the American College of Obstetricians and Gynecologists (ACOG) recommend that pregnant women go through the full term of their pregnancy before giving birth to ensure that their babies are fully developed. ACOG says unequivocally that elective deliveries with no medical indication from thirty-seven to thirty-nine weeks are unacceptable medical practice, but doctors have too often ignored this advice. Thousands of babies are delivered early each year without medical necessity and before the brain and other organs are fully developed.

Now, conscientious doctors and hospitals are reducing early elective deliveries. Physicians in the twenty largest hospitals in Ohio, for example, were asked to document a medical reason every time a woman was scheduled to deliver before thirty-nine weeks. In less than fifteen months, early deliveries without medical necessity plummeted. The number of babies admitted to neonatal intensive care dropped too, saving unnecessary heartache for parents. Revenue is falling at some hospitals because infants no longer need intensive care.

The entitlement mindset surfaced when executives at a hospital on the West Coast insisted that local employers pay the hospital for the one to two million dollars it was losing in revenue when it reduced early deliveries that were medically inappropriate. The request provoked a firestorm among businesses unaccustomed to working with a sense of entitlement to revenue. Most firms have to earn money by providing a high-quality product or service. Not so in health care.

An entitlement mindset nurtured for decades is hard to change. In this case, employers could make a reasonable argument that the hospital should reimburse them and their employees for the extra cost it billed them for all the medically inappropriate deliveries it performed over the years. This commonsense justice is unlikely to prevail. Hospitals know they have a monopoly on a service that anyone, at any moment, might need that could make the difference between life and death.

TOLERATES POOR PERFORMANCE

Hospitals do a lot of good. They are also places where a lot of preventable harm occurs. Large numbers of seniors on Medicare are harmed in hospitals each year because of medical errors, hospital-acquired infections, substandard care, and lack of proper monitoring, according to the Office of the Inspector General (OIG) in the U.S. Department of Health and Human Services.

About 79,200 Medicare beneficiaries a year experience a preventable error or other event that contributes to their deaths, according to an analysis conducted by the OIG. This number does not include preventable deaths in nursing homes, dialysis centers, and other settings where older Americans receive care. California, Florida, and New York are the top three states with the highest number of deaths: 7,985, 5,633, and 5,000, respectively, as shown in table 11.1. The hospital industry responded with deafening silence.

What happens when seniors are harmed, and who helps them? Do they go back to the hospital where they were harmed? Who speaks for them when they are too afraid, sick, or unfamiliar with medical care to know what to do?

Table 11.1. Annual Number of Medicare Beneficiaries Who Experience a Preventable Medical Mistake in a Hospital That Contributes to their Death, by State

State	# of Medicare Beneficiaries	State	# of Medicare Beneficiaries
Alabama	1,416	Nebraska	465
Alaska	108	Nevada	598
Arizona	1,550	New Hampshire	367
Arkansas	891	New Jersey	2,221
California	7,985	New Mexico	526
Colorado	1,048	New York	5,000
Connecticut	948	North Carolina	2,501
Delaware	250	North Dakota	180
District of Columbia	131	Ohio	3,172
Florida	5,633	Oklahoma	1,009
Georgia	2,086	Oregon	1,039
Hawaii	348	Pennsylvania	3,805
Idaho	386	Rhode Island	304
Illinois	3,080	South Carolina	1,302
Indiana	1,685	South Dakota	228
Iowa	863	Tennessee	1,773
Kansas	723	Texas	5,058
Kentucky	1,275	Utah	476
Louisiana	1,150	Vermont	187
Maine	443	Virginia	1,919
Maryland	1,319	Washington	1,633
Massachusetts	1,774	West Virginia	636
Michigan	2,773	Wisconsin	1,525
Minnesota	1,315	Wyoming	134
Mississippi	832	Guam, Puerto Rico, Virgin Islands	1,161
Missouri	1,677		
Montana	284	**Total**	**79,192**

Kathy Day, the nurse and patient safety activist in Maine, describes what happens when ordinary citizens are harmed and try to change policy for the public good:

> Patients are shunned. In fact, they are often subtly or sometimes cruelly blamed for their own harm, ignored, and rendered voiceless. Providers tend to sweep the events under the rug and not tell the patient. This erodes trust and is not conducive to improvement. Very little harm is reported, anywhere. That is why it is difficult for consumers to "shop" for the best and safest health care. Insiders know who are the most competent providers and who they would want caring for them or their loved ones. Everyone else is left to decide for themselves.

The public voice of conscientious citizens, endeavoring to hold health care accountable and make the mayhem stop, is muzzled. The citizen who wishes to participate in democracy is allowed to enter only the anteroom, if at all, outside the corridors of power where the decisions are made. Even then, citizens are invited in on the terms set by the powerbrokers. They are outsiders in their own country, whose so-called democracy is barely a shadow of what Thomas Jefferson and the signers of the Declaration of Independence had in mind.

The implicit message is that the public has to live with whatever is offered and be grateful. An attempt to craft legislation to hold hospitals accountable is met with the response that "you just don't understand" how health care works, notwithstanding evidence by conscientious physicians and nurses that irrefutably shows that so much harm is preventable.

Social stigma doesn't accrue to hospitals and other places where harm occurs. That's because hospitals save lives and improve the quality of life for so many people. Nevertheless, preventable harm is never excusable.

RESISTS SCRUTINY

The federal government does not release the names of hospitals that have the worst track records for patient harm. Hammering away at the secrecy in health care are public-interest advocacy organizations and journalists such as Consumers Union, Public Citizen, the Leapfrog Group, and ProPublica. The wall of silence has cracks now. For instance, hospitals are required to report central-line bloodstream infections in their intensive care units, one of the most deadly types of infections that causes about one-third of the nearly one hundrd thousand infection-related hospital deaths each year. Medicare posts the hospital infection information on its website.

Medicare officials and enlightened members of Congress launched a merit-based approach to paying hospitals, beginning with a common-sense, long-overdue policy to stop paying hospitals for medical mistakes such as wrong-site surgery or surgery on the wrong patient. A no-pay rule was adopted for certain infections that people acquire while they are in the hospital.

Beginning October 2012, Medicare started to give hospitals an incentive payment for how well they provide care for people with heart attacks, heart failure, and pneumonia and for people who have surgery. Hospitals will lose up to 1 percent of their annual increase if they don't achieve certain levels of performance. The stakes get higher with a loss of up to 2 percent in 2017. Hospitals can earn the money back by meeting performance targets.

A performance-based payment system is the right direction for public policy. Still, Medicare continues to pay for countless other causes of preventable health care harm, including those that contribute to the deaths of nearly eighty thousand seniors every year. That's because the hospital industry has so many resources for lobbying. Lisa McGiffert, director of the Safe Patient Project at Consumers Union, says the lobbying "drowns out consumers and sets up barriers every step of the way. The industry rarely calls out the worst of its members, so the public doesn't know which hospitals cause the most harm."

HAS REPUTATIONAL IMMUNITY

When illness strikes, nothing is more satisfying than to be cared for by a doctor who is competent. Competent doctors are self-motivated to keep their skills honed and knowledge up to date. They recognize that their medical school education and residency training are only the beginning of a lifelong commitment to continuous learning. Not content with being average, they are masters in their field and willing to have their competence assessed by objective third parties.

At the other end of the spectrum are doctors who are incompetent. Up to 12 percent of doctors are in this category, according to studies conducted by physicians about their peers.

Medicare does not discriminate between competent and incompetent doctors. It pays incompetent doctors as well as the competent ones. Medicare relies on the medical profession to determine who is competent. Unfortunately, the profession does a very poor job weeding out the incompetent doctors.

Why are incompetent doctors allowed to practice medicine? There are two reasons. First, when a state medical board grants a medical license, a doctor can practice for more than forty years and never be required to demonstrate that he or she is competent. State licensing boards do not require doctors to undergo any rigorous competency assessment as a condition of renewing their medical license every few years.

Five states—Colorado, Indiana, Montana, New York, and South Dakota—have no requirements that doctors keep up to date on medical knowledge, a far lower threshold than requiring doctors to demonstrate that they are competent.

When a public-interest-minded executive director of a medical board from one of these states proposed minimal continuing education requirements to renew a medical license, the state medical society protested vehemently to state legislators. The medical board director backed down under the threat of losing his job.

Most other states have requirements that doctors must meet to renew their license, but they are minimal in relation to the importance of the work doctors do. Doctors may need to complete continuing medical education requirements, which can be easily done by attending conferences.

Why are doctors allowed to practice with minimal oversight? The medical profession has established for itself reputational immunity. It is best characterized by a doctor who quipped about his colleagues, "There is a culture of independence. . . . Once I'm finished with my education I'm a law unto myself."

Once a doctor has been granted a medical license by the state licensing board, it becomes an entitlement that many doctors keep for the remainder of their lives. State medical boards have been known to renew the licenses of doctors even when they are retired and no longer provide care to patients. Doctors say their personal and professional lives are intertwined, and a medical license is part of their identity.

Courts have ruled that a medical license is a property right in cases of divorce. In a landmark case, the New York Court of Appeals ruled, "A professional license is a valuable property right, reflected in the money, effort and lost opportunity for employment expended in its acquisition, and also in the enhanced earning capacity it affords its holder, which may not be revoked without due process of law." Unfortunately for the public, the fact that a medical license is a property right to generate private gain often trumps the reality that it is also a license granted by the state where the doctor practices to serve the public's interest.

Doctors may choose to have their knowledge reassessed periodically and have aspects of their practice be objectively examined by a third party by gaining, and maintaining, certification by a specialty board in medicine such as the American Board of Surgery or the American Board of Family Medicine. The requirements to maintain board certification are more rigorous than to maintain a medical license and have been strengthened in the past decade.

Nonetheless, these requirements are not nearly as stringent as those of other professions whose competence affects public safety. A trenchant and revealing analysis by two doctors, Donald Trunkey and Richard Botney, compared how doctors and airline pilots are assessed in a landmark article, "Assessing Competency: A Tale of Two Professions." Unlike doctors, airline pilots must pass rigorous performance examinations every year. During unannounced inspections conducted by the Federal Aviation Administration, which grants pilot licenses, skills are assessed on-site in the cockpit. Commercial airline carriers that employ pilots perform their own separate on-site assessments in the cockpit. Pilots must obtain a first-class medical certificate every six months. The medical evaluation includes neurologic and psychiatric evaluations. Pilots are required to submit to random drug tests. Doctors are not subject to any comparable performance assessment or medical evaluation.

Doctors are accorded reputational immunity because they have specialized knowledge that lay persons do not have. Those who are not competent are protected by membership in a club that confers immunity from scrutiny. Lobbying and campaign contributions to politicians seeking elective office solidify reputation immunity.

Licenses are rarely revoked for incompetence. The watchdog group Public Citizen reported that the number of doctors disciplined by state medical boards has declined 20 percent between 2004 and 2010. The rare exceptions when doctors are disciplined usually involve cases of drug and sex abuse. Even in these cases, the wheels of public protection move slowly.

When a medical board suspends a doctor's license to practice medicine or otherwise disciplines a doctor, the reaction can prompt retaliation indicative of an entitlement mindset. In Arkansas in 2009, a doctor who had his license revoked by the state medical board placed a grenade near the car owned by the executive director of the board, Dr. Trent Pierce. When Dr. Pierce turned on the ignition, the device exploded. He suffered serious injuries to his face and body, and he lost sight in his left eye and hearing in his left ear. After a massive investigation by authorities, the perpetrator was identified, charged, and sentenced to prison. Dr. Pierce resumed his duties with the medical board after months of treatment and recovery.

A less harrowing form of retaliation occurred when the executive director of a state medical board in the Northeast received verbal threats and animal carcasses in the mail from doctors the board sanctioned. The director requested and received security protection from the state police. An executive director of a state medical board in the Midwest was verbally assaulted and received threats to her career from the colleague of a physician who had been disciplined by the board for failure to comply with state license requirements.

Public Citizen called on the federal government to investigate state medical boards for their failure to protect seniors on Medicare from doctors who are an immediate risk to their health and safety. It reported that 220 physicians were considered by the hospitals or managed care plans where they worked to be an immediate threat to the public. Seventy-five percent of them were stripped of their clinical privileges on an emergency basis, meaning they were no longer permitted to work in those facilities. Yet state medical boards took no action, and the doctors continue to have a medical license and can practice somewhere else.

The Office of the Inspector General in the U.S. Department of Health and Human Services can exclude a doctor from participating in the Medicare program if a threat to seniors' health exists and when a state medical board fails to act. The public can access names of doctors who have been excluded from providing care to seniors on Medicare in an online searchable database. Here is an example cited by Public Citizen where the federal government was compelled to act when a state medical board did not:

> The OIG excluded a California oncologist for 10 years . . . because the OIG determined that he had rendered over 3,900 excessive, substandard, unnecessary, and potentially risky services to seven Medicare beneficiaries over a six year period of time. . . . Once the exclusion was in place, the licensing board did revoke the doctor's license. Then it stayed the revocation and put the license on probation. The stay has been lifted but if the OIG had not devoted its investigative power . . . to excluding this physician, the Medicare . . . patient population would have continued to be at grave risk during the four years that the licensing board took to get to an exclusionable point in its process.

Republican senators Charles Grassley from Iowa and Orrin Hatch from Utah and Democrat Max Baucus from Montana shined a spotlight on instances where physicians were sanctioned by their employer for wrongdoing, including sexual misconduct and fraud, but kept their medical license. They asked the Office of the Inspector General in the Department of Health and Human Services to evaluate state medical boards' performance. So far the OIG has not done so. The likely impediment is pressure from the medical lobby to protect its members from unwelcome scrutiny.

BREEDS CORRUPTION

Arthur Brooks, president of the conservative Washington think tank, the American Enterprise Institute, described the "malignant cronyism" that plagues America in an opinion editorial in the *Wall Street Journal*. He wrote, "The Occupy Wall Street movement was at least right to protest the malignant cronyism in our economy."

The same malignant cronyism is alive and well in health care. One of the most costly examples is the two-hundred-billion-dollar market where hospital supplies and equipment are bought and sold. Hospitals and other health care providers typically use middlemen known as group purchasing organizations (GPOs) to buy supplies such as Band-Aids and medical devices such as defibrillators and hip implants. A handful of GPOs divide up about 90 percent of the market.

Manufacturers and vendors that want to sell their products to hospitals through these purchasing organizations pay them fees up to 3 percent of sales volume. In return, they gain access to customers that buy billions of dollars of supplies and equipment. They also gain control over the products that hospitals purchase.

GPOs used to be like Costco, which receives dues from members and buys products wholesale from manufacturers at the lowest price and passes the savings on to members. That changed in 1986 when Congress granted GPOs an exemption from Medicare's antikickback laws, which unleashed a polished form of legal white-collar corruption.

GPOs' main source of revenue changed from hospitals to manufacturers of supplies, equipment, and drugs. If GPOs negotiate with a manufacturer for a lower price for antibacterial soap, for instance, their revenue will decline. So GPOs have an incentive to favor companies that sell the highest-price products and pay the largest fees.

In a classic monopoly, a GPO might sign a single-source contract with a manufacturer or vendor and receive a bonus for doing so. As with any monopoly, single-source contacts drive up prices and lock out companies that offer better products at lower prices.

Companies locked out of the market have sued and won. A jury awarded more than five hundred million dollars in damages against a manufacturer of hospital beds that used GPO contracts to exclude a competitor from the market.

The Department of Justice has investigated GPOs for allegations of anticompetitive behavior and kickbacks, but federal authorities have taken no action against a GPO in nearly a decade. Lawmakers in Congress and executive branch officials have protected the GPOs even though price transparency and competition at the wholesale level would save Medicare billions of dollars. Government-proffered privilege breeds corruption and undermines the integrity of a vital supply chain in the health care industry.

A trenchant analysis of GPOs alleges that they wield so much power that they, not clinicians, decide the drugs, devices, and supplies used in the hospitals.

If hospitals don't buy enough volume, they pay stiff financial penalties. These arrangements may explain why the Midwest surgeon who reviewed the inventory in his operating room discovered excess supplies. To avoid big penalties, a hospital will purchase more than it needs.

Fraud in Medicare takes many other forms. As a former Medicare official explained to us, there are two kinds of Medicare fraud. The first type is perpetrated by criminal gangs. The government's fraud reduction is targeted largely at criminal gangs because the political cost is much lower. Low-level gangs don't have lobbyists.

The second type is white-collar fraud carried out by drug companies, device manufacturers, hospitals, doctors, hospices, dialysis facilities, and other providers. White-collar fraud is pursued much more delicately because the fraudsters may be well connected in the White House or Congress. Run-of-the-mill fraud turns into corruption when protected by government officials. A handful of white-collar cases might be prosecuted each year to give the public the impression that the federal government is tough on fraud. Corporate cases rarely name top executives and companies never admit wrongdoing. Fines are a small blip on the balance sheet. Federal investigators avoid treading on politically protected territory because a phone call can stop an investigation in its tracks. Both kinds of fraud consume 10 percent of Medicare spending, or nearly sixty billion dollars a year.

Financial finagling also occurs under the category of "improper payments." These are mistakes made because of errors in calculating payment. They are not considered fraud because of the absence of intent to deceive for inappropriate gain, or at least the absence of evidence to prove intent to defraud. Medicare made forty-eight billion dollars in improper payments in 2010. These payments also include those made without adequate documentation of the medical necessity for surgery or other treatments, which presents abundant opportunity for mischief.

A more mundane but rampant type of abuse occurred as we were writing this book. An organization that called itself American Seniors Assistance called one of us and asked if any seniors on Medicare lived in the house, and if so, did they have diabetes and arthritis. Sensing a scam and desiring to learn firsthand how Medicare is being abused, the reply was yes, a fictional older woman lived in the house and she had arthritis.

The caller asked if the senior had lower back pain and knee pain and offered to have a back brace and knee braces delivered to the house by mail that "will help the arthritis in her back and knees," and "all doctors are recommending it" at "no cost" to the senior. Then the caller inquired whether the fictional senior has trouble getting up from a sofa, and the response was once again, yes. He said he will send a seat assist that looks like a small pillow. By pressing a button, it rises and supposedly helps an older person stand up.

To place an order, the caller wanted the name of the Medicare beneficiary. Being reluctant to give even fictional information to a stranger, the request was made to know more about the organization. The representative said he was a volunteer and worked at a nonprofit organization. When asked to speak with a manager, the caller said his manager was busy. This abuse was reported to the Medicare fraud hotline, which documented the information.

In a surprising finding, government corruption is not far from the minds of Americans. When a Gallup poll asked Americans during the run-up to the 2012 presidential campaign what the priorities should be for the next president, nearly half of Americans—45 percent—said that corruption in the federal government is an extremely important concern. In an interview on *Marketplace*, Frank Newport, the editor-in-chief at Gallup, said that Americans are "very, very negative about their federal government and the way congress is working." Most Americans don't think about Medicare and corruption in the same sentence. They should.

SILENCES CRITICS

We have the honor of knowing a very talented physician who led a team of researchers that studied the effects of a drug used to help people cope with a life-threatening disease. The drug was widely advertised on television. He and his team discovered a startling finding: the drug accelerated progression of the disease. People who dutifully consumed it were unwittingly taking slow poison.

The findings were irrefutable and published in a well-known medical journal. Doctors stopped using the drug, sales plummeted, and the FDA issued warnings. The doctor and his research team performed an immense public service.

By exposing the truth, a small empire crashed. The well-known drug company that manufactured and marketed the drug lost a multi-billion-dollar blockbuster that turned out to be a killer. As drug company revenue dried up, employees lost jobs. The average house value in the community where they lived dropped by a hundred housand dollars. Advertising agency employees who created the ads for the killer drug lost their jobs.

In return for his service to humanity, well-funded special interests whose entitlement was cut off tried to derail the doctor's career. They circulated false rumors to his colleagues and neighbors. He was forced out of a prestigious teaching and research position, leaving behind millions of dollars in research funding that he obtained based on his track record and expertise. He moved far away to a new place of employment to rebuild his professional career. He worries whether he can afford to send his children to college.

Rather than celebrate the truth, an entitlement-based industry sees truth as the enemy. The company sought to destroy the messenger with a ruthlessness that is a hidden reality of health care today. No one speaks about it publicly. It is whispered during coffee breaks at medical meetings.

The American Medical Association should close ranks and protect members of the profession who perform an important public service, but it doesn't. If a president of a physician organization proposed to take this moral high ground, he would be fired and have trouble landing another job.

Many doctors have individually and collectively become agents of the industry rather than agents of their patients. If they worked in the sphere of foreign affairs, they would be labeled double agents. If they sold out to the highest bidder and betrayed the people for whom they were obliged to work, it would be called treason.

The new generation of doctors will not know what it is like to practice medicine without the corrupting influence of multibillion-dollar drug and device manufacturers that work diligently to hide, manipulate, and destroy the truth in slavish devotion to a profit imperative.

SEEKS PROTECTION FROM THE POLITICAL ELITE

Elite capture occurs when influential individuals and businesses, by virtue of money and stature, change government policy to suit their interests. Here is an example.

The National Practitioner Data Bank contains the names of doctors and other health care professionals who have paid malpractice claims or have been disciplined by a hospital or licensing board. It is maintained by the Health Resources and Services Administration (HRSA) in the Department of Health and Human Services. Hospitals and managed-care organizations use the data bank to check the backgrounds of people before they hire them. A public-use file allowed journalists and researchers to have access to the information. Names and addresses of doctors and other health care professionals were kept confidential.

In fall 2011, Alan Bavley, a reporter from the *Kansas City Star,* wrote a story about a Kansas doctor, Robert Tenny, who had been sued at least sixteen times for malpractice and had paid nearly $3.7 million in claims in the past twenty years. Bavley was writing about doctors with a trail of alleged malpractice who have not been disciplined by the Kansas medical board.

The doctor contacted HRSA and alleged that the journalist violated the rules of confidentiality when using information from the data bank. In fact, the reporter had acted lawfully. He used the data bank's public-access files and combined the information with other publicly available information to identify the doctor.

Under pressure from the doctor and his lawyer, federal government staff threatened the reporter with civil penalties. Also, they shut down public access to information in the data bank.

Senator Charles Grassley wrote to Health and Human Services Secretary Kathleen Sebelius criticizing the move, saying,

> The intent of the legislation that created the Public Use File was to . . . restrict the ability of incompetent healthcare practitioners to relocate without discovery of previous substandard performance or unprofessional conduct. However, from the documents provided by HRSA it appears that instead of protecting the interest of public health, its purpose was to protect a single physician who had a malpractice suit and disciplinary action filed against him. Instead of conducting its own research into the professional conduct of Dr. Tenny, HRSA appears to have overreacted to the complaint of a single physician based on no evidence other than that he received a call from the press.

The Association of Health Care Journalists and other organizations wrote to the Department of Health and Human Services objecting to the shutdown, saying they need access to information in the data bank to expose failures in states' regulatory enforcement that have caused harm to patients. "As a result of these stories, states have enacted new legislation and medical boards have taken steps to investigate problem doctors," said Charles Ornstein, president of the journalists' group.

Under mounting pressure from public-interest advocates and Senator Grassley, HRSA agreed to reinstate public access but imposed onerous restrictions. Journalists must agree that they won't use the information with other data sources to identify any of the 196,000 doctors with a record of a malpractice or disciplinary action. These restrictions prevent journalists like Alan Bavley from reporting on doctors who pose a risk to the health and safety of the public.

Here is what Bavley uncovered and subsequently wrote in the *Kansas City Star* about the impact of the new restrictions:

> Buried deep in a federal database is Practitioner No. 222117, perhaps the most frequently disciplined doctor in America. This doctor has been accused of violating drug laws, prescribing unauthorized medications, providing substandard care and obtaining licenses through fraud. From 2002 through 2006, 20 states and the District of Columbia revoked or suspended No. 222117's medical licenses. Two professional societies took away the doctor's memberships. The Department of Health and Human Services banned the doctor from billing Medicare and Medicaid. And the Drug Enforcement Administration revoked the doctor's permit to prescribe controlled drugs. For most of these years, the doctor's home base was Missouri.

Bavley reported that the federal government won't let anyone know who this doctor is even though he or she is a clear threat to the public's health. In the past, journalists who combed court records and state medical board actions might have been able to piece together the identity of medical scofflaws, but now they are prevented from doing so.

Other doctors in the National Practitioner Data Bank who pose a threat to the public's health include a surgeon who lost or settled 247 malpractice cases in California during the 1990s, and a doctor with drug and alcohol problems for the past twenty years who has been the subject of actions by hospitals and licensing boards in at least five states.

The overwhelming majority of Americans—nine in ten—say the public should have access to information about doctors who have a sketchy track record, according to a *Consumer Reports* poll. But now they have less information to make more informed choices.

The medical profession seeks protection from the political elite to curb rightful scrutiny on matters affecting public health and safety. Those seeking protection may be the least deserving of a medical license and protection from public scrutiny.

In the end, one doctor shut down lawful access to vital public information. That's entitlement.

· 12 ·

Hedge Funds: The Newest
Beneficiaries of Medicare's Entitlement

*W*hat happens when you bring together the son of a famous U.S. senator and hedge funds? Hedge fund principals and their clients receive VIP access to high-level Washington officials whose decisions regarding Medicare affect the rise and fall of stocks and other investments the funds buy and sell on Wall Street.

That's exactly what happened when the Marwood Company, whose president is Ted Kennedy Jr., son of the late Senator Edward Kennedy of Massachusetts, orchestrated a meeting with hedge fund analysts and Medicare officials.

The New York–based Marwood touts its services to institutional investors, health care corporations, and trade associations. Its unique role is to give investors and operators in the health care industry "a deep understanding of the complex rules and regulations that can impact business goals," it says on its website. The firm is peppered with members of the Kennedy clan, including Robert F. Kennedy Jr., who serves as an advisor, and it boasts about its employees who come from the ranks of the White House, Congress, and Medicare.

For Senator Ted Kennedy, who died of a brain tumor in 2009, universal health insurance coverage was "the cause" of his life. Kennedy's son has been helping industry players maximize their bottom lines by giving them unique access to top government officials.

Marwood sought inside information on pending Medicare decisions that would affect its clients' investment decisions. The Project on Government Oversight (POGO), an independent watchdog that investigates government corruption, misconduct, and conflicts of interest, reported on a meeting set up by Marwood with top Medicare officials. A whistleblower who worked in the Medicare agency filed an ethics complaint about the special access given to a select group of Wall Street operators.

The whistleblower said that about a dozen Medicare officials participated in a two-hour briefing with Wall Street operatives eager to ferret out information about whether Medicare was planning to pay for new medical devices for seniors. Medicare's decision could have far-reaching consequences for the value of their investments.

"They got to probe us for hours in private about what we planned to do and how we approached procedures for reimbursing medical devices, the mechanics and psychology of decision-making in general and with respect to these specific devices," the whistleblower told POGO.

No allegations were made that Medicare officials profited personally from the meetings or that inside information was disclosed. But high-level government officials had to spend time, paid by taxpayers, answering questions posed by Wall Street twentysomethings seeking to gather information to help them identify hot stocks to buy and other stocks to sell. Meetings such as this one were routine practice, the whistleblower told us.

Armed with as much information as they can glean, Wall Street operators can hail a taxi from the Department of Health and Human Services on Independence Avenue and arrive on Capitol Hill in minutes to meet with influential members of Congress and encourage them to put in a good word to Medicare to make a decision favorable to their investors.

The whistleblower was fired for being disloyal to the agency mission. The ethics office in the Medicare agency found no inappropriate use of government employees' time.

We spoke with the whistleblower and concluded that if the American public had the opportunity to judge this person by society's norms, not Washington's norms, they would conclude that the whistleblower was a true public servant who has only the public's interest in mind.

The whistleblower described how the culture of government service has changed as the influence of special interests has permeated every nook and cranny in Washington. Fifty years ago, many public-spirited citizens went to work in Washington to serve the country, inspired by President John Kennedy's urging for Americans to "ask not what your country can do for you. Ask what you can do for your country."

Today, the mantra for those who profit excessively from Medicare has become, "What can my country do for me." Federal employees who want to act for the public's benefit face Berlin Wall–like roadblocks set up by special interests, who try to manipulate government decisions to increase their private gain.

SEISMIC SHIFTS IN MEDICARE IMPERCEPTIBLE TO THE PUBLIC

If highly qualified public officials who work for Medicare determine that the best scientific evidence shows that a device or drug would harm seniors, and they recommend that Medicare should not pay for it, the company that makes the product will lobby higher-ups to overturn the recommendation.

If Medicare staff build a solid case against a company for defrauding billions of dollars from Medicare by providing defective equipment that could place seniors in harm's way, but the company is politically well connected with the White House or senators, the Justice Department will be told to back down and not prosecute the case.

Most Americans understand that lobbyists influence Washington policy makers. Today, lobbyists do much more than that. They set the rules and ensure that Congress and the White House enforce them. The industry has routine contact with congressional staff, officials in the Department of Health and Human Services, and White House advisors. Their own handpicked people are hired in the federal government to make certain that decisions are made in their favor.

Medicare is a pot of gold for drug companies, device manufacturers, hospitals, and other businesses. Because so much money is in play, Medicare's mission has been hijacked by the medical-industrial complex. Ostensibly, Medicare officials' primary accountability is to seniors and the public. In reality, the outsized influence of the industry in Washington has shifted the accountability of government to big-moneyed interests. It is enormously challenging for public-spirited civil servants and elected officials to do the work the public pays them to do. The cumulative impact of decades of marriage between the businesses that believe they are entitled to excessive amounts of Medicare money and their enabling entitlers has created a Medicare program that is very different from the one envisioned by its creators.

When the OIG reported that nearly eighty thousand seniors a year on Medicare die because of failures in hospital safety, patient safety advocates and family members who lost parents or grandparents would have been eager to meet with high-level Medicare officials and grill them for two hours on how Medicare could let that number of seniors succumb to blatantly bad treatment. Lacking money and an army of lobbyists to open doors to decision makers and directly influence public policy, they will never get in the door.

Some Democrats don't want the public to hear this message because it undercuts the belief of many progressives that government is the solution. The pervasiveness of elite capture may drive some people to believe that vouchers might be a better answer because they would privatize Medicare and take government out of the picture. This is not a solution either, because the insurance industry will become even more powerful with millions more enrollees.

HOW WALL STREET CASHED IN ON HEALTH CARE REFORM

During the health care reform debate, one of the most contentious issues was whether the uninsured would be covered by insurance provided by a public program similar to Medicare or by private health insurance. The health insurance industry vehemently opposed the public option because it would lose the chance to have sixteen million newly insured customers who would be required to buy a product from one of its companies to comply with the individual mandate.

Hedge funds wanted inside information to know how Congress would vote on the public option in December 2009. If Congress okayed the public option, health insurance company stocks would plummet. If the public option was defeated, private insurance stock prices would jump.

Instead of waiting to find out how Congress would vote on the public option, as ordinary investors would have to do, big-money Wall Street operators wanted the information before anyone else. If the public option was slated for defeat, they would buy stock in insurance companies, betting that the price would rise after the vote was announced. If the public option were to prevail, they could dump their shares of private insurance company stocks and minimize their losses.

Hedge funds found a company that would help them get ahead of the information curve. According to the *Wall Street Journal*, JNK Securities helped hedge fund clients gain access to key senators who were likely to cast the deciding Senate votes on the public option. Senator Joseph Lieberman from Connecticut was one of them. Connecticut is the home state of Aetna, which sells health insurance. Lieberman told *Face the Nation* about his stance on the public option: "I think it's such a mistake that I would use the power I have as a single Senator to stop a final vote."

According to the company's website, JNK offers "real time intelligence on all matters of US government policy." It arranges one-on-one meetings with key stakeholders, roundtable discussions, meetings, and conference calls but doesn't lobby for legislation or raise money for political campaigns.

True to its advertisement, JNK Securities arranged a meeting with hedge fund clients Viking Global and Karsch Capital, Senator Lieberman, and other key legislators shortly before the Senate voted on the public option, the *Wall Street Journal* reported. Lieberman's staff spokesperson said that the senator does not give any special information to one group that he wouldn't share with any other group, constituent, or the media.

The Senate voted down the public insurance option, boosting the outlook for private health insurers. During the fourth quarter of 2009, Viking Global bought six million shares of Aetna stock, and Karsch bought half a million Aetna shares during the same period, according to regulatory records reviewed by *Journal* reporters.

Since March 2010, when President Obama signed health care reform into law, health insurance company stocks have had a good run. Almost two and a half years later, Aetna's stock price had gained 18 percent, Cigna climbed 22 percent, and UnitedHealthcare enjoyed a 72 percent rise.

POLITICAL INTELLIGENCE: GOOD OR BAD?

Political intelligence is the fuel that runs Washington. Policy makers need information to craft and enact legislation that serves the public's interest.

Wall Streeters do what they are good at doing. They create markets. They created a market for exclusive political intelligence in Washington. Clients who want information pay handsomely for it. Government officials supply the information. Brokers set up meetings where information is transacted behind closed doors.

Investors want to be ahead of the information curve so they can act in the market before anyone else, reaping a financial advantage. The exclusivity of trading in political information for private financial gain is the distinguishing and disturbing feature of this market. Moneyed interests buy access to information that is not available to people without money or access. It provides more proof to Americans who are busy going about their daily lives that the system is rigged for the benefit of a few at their expense. Government officials spend time paid for by taxpayers to give special attention to Wall Street insiders whose sole purpose is private gain.

The market for political intelligence has changed the landscape where Medicare's future will be decided. The political playing field is stacked against the interests of seniors, boomers, and everyone who pays for Medicare and will depend on it one day. Official Washington has forgotten who it works for. That can never be good for hardworking people who desperately want a government they can trust.

HOW PUBLIC OUTRAGE CURBED THE WORST ABUSES

Public outrage hit a high point when *60 Minutes* reported in 2012 that members of Congress traded stocks using insider information they received while carrying out their public duties. Peter Schweizer, author of *Throw Them All Out*, documented the stock trades of members of Congress and investigated who bought and sold drug stocks during the debate on the Medicare prescription drug legislation in 2003.

Senator John Kerry, a Democrat from Massachusetts, and his wife, the heiress to the Heinz ketchup fortune, were the biggest insider traders. Kerry's committee in the Senate had oversight of the Medicare Part D drug bill, and he was familiar with the legislation.

According to Kerry's 2003 financial disclosure statements, he and his wife made 111 stock transactions, and 103 of them were purchases of stocks of drug companies and health insurers. In September 2003 when the legislation was being crafted, they made nine purchases of drug maker Johnson & Johnson totaling five hundred thousand dollars and sixteen purchases of Pfizer stock worth one million dollars. When the bill became law, drug company stock prices jumped. Kerry and his wife sold some of their drug stocks and made thousands of dollars in gains. Kerry went on to become the 2004 presidential nominee of the Democratic party.

Not everyone took advantage of insider information, according to Schweizer. James Sensenbrenner, a Republican member of the House of Representatives from Wisconsin who owned millions of dollars in drug stocks, didn't trade during the debate on Medicare drug coverage.

The biggest player in the health care industry who operated on both sides of the fence simultaneously was Bill Frist, a former Republican senator from Tennessee first elected in 1994. Frist became Senate majority leader in 2003, a post he held until he left the Senate in January 2007.

In Medicare's infancy in the mid-1960s, Bill Frist's father, Thomas Frist Sr., started the Hospital Corporation of America (HCA), which is now the largest for-profit hospital company in the country. Two years after Frist arrived in the Senate, HCA was investigated for Medicare fraud and later settled with the government for $1.7 billion in fines.

During his time on Capitol Hill, Frist was hounded by public-interest advocates who claimed that although he had no formal role with HCA, his close family ties to the company and his wealth that derived from HCA could give, at best, the appearance of a conflict of interest. The watchdog group Common Cause asked the Senate ethics committee to reconsider whether Frist should be allowed to vote on bills that would help his family's business. Nothing came of its effort.

Frist served on the Senate Finance Committee Subcommittee on Health and the Committee on Health, Education, Labor, and Pensions. Frist pushed for legislation to limit jury awards in medical malpractice cases. The legislation would have helped a subsidiary of HCA, Health Care Indemnity, one of the country's largest providers of medical malpractice insurance, by limiting its payouts for negligence. Another public interest group, Consumer Watchdog, wrote to Frist urging him to recuse himself from voting and advocating for the bill, saying,

> Senate financial disclosures reveal that you and your immediate family own at least $25 million in HCA stock and your inheritance is

clearly dependent on the success of the financial fortunes of the company. HCA and its doctors will benefit from any limits on liability
for malpractice, however, the pork for the company in the legislation
you are hurrying to the floor Tuesday is beyond the pale. You should
immediately recuse yourself from pending votes on liability caps, end
your personal advocacy . . . and abstain from any future involvement
in the medical malpractice debate. . . . You have failed to explain
why your actions, which would increase your family fortune, your
own investments and perhaps your inheritance, are not a conflict of
interest. Never has the need for you to step aside been more clear.

Frist responded to allegations of conflict of interest by saying that
his assets were in a blind trust and not under his active control. Blind
trusts are designed to be a firewall between federal officials and their
investments so they don't enrich themselves by using their elected office.

Federal investigators set their sights on Frist in early June 2005
when he directed the trustees of his blind trust to sell shares of HCA.
A month later the stock price had the biggest decline in more than two
years because of warnings that earnings would not meet Wall Street
expectations. By that time, Frist's shares had been sold. The Department
of Justice and the Securities and Exchange Commission investigated
whether Frist had used insider information when he ordered the trade.
Frist was the first congressional leader to be formally investigated by federal authorities for insider stock trading. He contended that he engaged
in no wrongdoing and used publicly available information. Shareholders
are not allowed to use insider information to buy and sell stock. If Frist
had been found to have traded stocks using information from his rela-
tives, he could have been convicted under the Securities Exchange Act.

Frist did not seek reelection for his Senate seat in the 2006 Republican primary. In November 2006 he announced that he would not run
for president. That same month, Frist's brother, Thomas Frist Jr., took
HCA private with the help of private-equity firms that included Bain
Capital and Kohlberg Kravis Roberts.

The SEC closed its investigation the following year without any
charges being filed, and Frist was cleared of any wrongdoing. Later that
same year, Frist was hired as a partner and chairman of the executive
board of private investment firm Cressey and Company, which special-
izes in health care.

The lesson is that one of the highest-ranking officials in the U.S. government, along with his family, had an enormous financial stake in the health care industry. Yet he continued to play a major role in health care legislation. Meanwhile, the fervent desire of ordinary Americans of all political stripes is to trust their elected officials beyond a shadow of a doubt.

In 2012 Bill Frist's brother, Thomas Frist Jr., was ranked by *Forbes* as the one hundred and twentieth richest billionaire in the United States, worth $3.2 billion.

Five months after *60 Minutes* aired the program on insider trading in Washington, Congress passed the STOCK Act, the Stop Trading on Congressional Knowledge Act. It prohibits members of Congress and their staff from using any nonpublic information obtained in the course of their duties, or by virtue of their position, for personal benefit. The bill applies to all employees in the executive and judicial branches of the federal government too.

Members of Congress are required to publicly disclose their transactions on their websites and file reports of any financial transaction of stocks, bonds, commodity futures, and other securities over one thousand dollars within forty-five days rather than once a year. Transactions by a member's spouse and children must also be disclosed. Special access to initial public stock offerings is prohibited. If violators are convicted of felonies involving public corruption, they are denied federal pensions. The law requires the Government Accountability Office to produce a report on the role of political intelligence firms in the financial markets.

Timely reporting makes it easier for watchdogs to link financial transactions to members' positions and votes on related issues. But will the STOCK Act change the culture of immunity? The law is no guarantee. It requires only the reporting of financial transactions. While the law may have a deterrent effect, it is only as strong as the political will to enforce it and prosecute some of the most powerful people in the country.

· 13 ·

The Entitlers:
The White House and Congress

$\mathcal{T}$he 2012 presidential campaign and the primaries leading up to it had a roster of candidates, many of whom had a track record during their political careers of being generous to the health care industry. Meanwhile, industry special interests lined up to preserve and protect the more than two trillion dollars that Medicare is projected to spend from 2013 to 2016—and which they will receive.

The health care industry put its money on President Obama to ensure that the Patient Protection and Affordable Care Act remained intact. Months before the November election, Obama garnered nearly seventeen million dollars from the health sector, according to the Center for Responsive Politics, the nonpartisan, nonprofit group that tracks political donations. The industry stands to gain a lot of money when up to thirty-two million newly insured people are added to its balance sheets.

Romney vowed to repeal the reform law, which caused industry donations to trail only slightly at fifteen million dollars. His campaign attracted a lot of cash from opponents of the health reform law within hours of the June 2012 U.S. Supreme Court ruling that upheld its constitutionality. More than forty-seven thousand donors contributed nearly five million dollars in just twenty-four hours.

That didn't stop the health insurance industry from writing checks for Romney's bid, acknowledging his running mate Paul Ryan, whose original Medicare proposal would have turned Medicare completely over to private health insurance plans, giving a big boost to the industry. Ryan pulled back from that plan, and the Republican National Convention platform called for continuing traditional Medicare for seniors. Still, Republicans have a track record of wanting to privatize Medicare.

Many of the early contenders for the Republican nomination had a history of receiving cash from the industry in return for serving as its benefactors using public money.

NEWT GINGRICH AND THE MEDICARE DRUG BENEFIT

Newt Gingrich, former speaker of the House of Representatives, has played an outsized role in shaping Medicare, notably in 2003 during the Medicare prescription drug debate, even though by that time he had left Congress. He urged fiscal conservatives to add a prescription drug benefit to the Medicare program. Gingrich was so enthusiastic that he penned an opinion editorial in the *Wall Street Journal* rallying fellow Republicans to vote in favor of the drug bill, stating in part:

> Although some conservatives may complain about the cost of the drug benefit, this benefit was designed within the framework of the budget resolution. The Medicare drug benefit is a necessary improvement to a Medicare system that was designed before modern pharmaceuticals became a key to staying healthy. . . .
>
> Conservatives now have a chance to pass a sound Medicare drug benefit that includes very significant improvements to the Medicare program. This bill has reforms . . . which will save lives and money. . . . Obstructionist conservatives can always find reasons to vote no, but that path leads right back into the minority and it would be a minority status they would deserve. . . . If you are a fiscal conservative who cares about balancing the federal budget, there may be no more important vote in your career than one in support of this bill.

During the Medicare drug debate, Gingrich was paid handsomely by drug company clients of his now-defunct health care firm, Center for Health Transformation. He gathered about two dozen Republican House members who did not support the Medicare prescription drug benefit to urge them to change their minds.

Fast-forward ten years and fiscal conservatives are fuming about the unfunded liabilities of Medicare Part D, which total sixteen trillion dollars, according to Medicare program actuaries. This figure is the amount of general revenues needed to pay for it in perpetuity. Gingrich has been critical of Medicare's third-party payer model that pays hospitals and doctors separately for each test and procedure, a wasteful practice, yet he espoused the new Medicare benefit that is the mother of all budget busters.

During his short-lived run for the Republican nomination for president in 2012, Gingrich was beholden to the health care industry, thanks to its deep pockets that shelled out thirty-seven million dollars over eight years to his firm. Top-brass contributors included the American Hospital Association, GE Medical, health insurer WellPoint, and drug company AstraZeneca.

RICK SANTORUM AND FOR-PROFIT HOSPITALS

Rick Santorum, the former senator from Pennsylvania and unsuccessful candidate for the 2012 Republican nomination, railed about Medicare being financially unsustainable. During the Iowa caucuses, Santorum said, "You have Medicare driving the entire health care system in this country and it's crushing it." One of the solutions he proposed on *Meet the Press* was means testing Medicare and requiring higher-income seniors to pay higher premiums.

Unknown to most voters, when he left the Senate after losing a reelection bid in 2006, Santorum became a board member of a for-profit hospital company based in King of Prussia, Pennsylvania, Universal Health Services (UHS). Santorum received $395,000 in director fees and stock options, according to the *New York Times*. While in the Senate, he sponsored legislation to increase Medicare payments to hospitals in Puerto Rico that would have added four hundred million dollars over ten years to Medicare spending. UHS owned hospitals in Puerto Rico and eventually sold them; it is uncertain whether it benefited.

When Santorum launched his presidential bid, he left the UHS board and reported between $100,001 and $250,000 in UHS stock. Company employees were the second top contributors to Santorum's campaign, donating twenty thousand dollars, according to data compiled by the Center for Responsive Politics. Employees at health insurer Blue Cross and Blue Shield were the top contributors, shelling out $22,750.

While Santorum was critical of Americans becoming dependent on government handouts, he wasn't critical of the companies he helped become more dependent on government.

RON PAUL AND CORPORATISM

Another Republican contender, Congressman Ron Paul from Texas, was more honest about corporate entitlements to Medicare. A practicing physician for many years, Paul said during the campaign that as president he would not immediately cut health care benefits for the elderly and children. He acknowledged his soft stance on Medicare in an interview with the *PBS NewsHour*, saying, "I haven't emphasized that at all."

Paul was one of the few candidates who was candid about the outsized role of big business in health care. "The most popular place to cut is the corporate welfare," he said during the interview. "Most of the money we spend in this country to help the poor is really helping the corporations. It is corporatism that is so bad whether it is medicine, or even in education or the military-industrial complex. The corporatism is the welfare that is huge."

JOHN HUNTSMAN AND DIALYSIS CENTERS

The former Republican governor of Utah and Ambassador to China in the Obama Administration, John Huntsman had a short-lived stint campaigning for the Republican nomination. Huntsman agreed with Paul Ryan's plan, saying, "Medicare won't be a sacred cow," and "across the board, I will tell the upper income category in this country that there will be means testing." His stance on taxes was, in part, to say "so long to corporate welfare and subsidies," although he wasn't explicit about subsidies to corporate health care.

One of the top contributors to Huntsman's campaign, Fresenius Medical Care, is the largest kidney dialysis company in the United States. It has its sights set on the huge business potential in China, where Huntsman was ambassador and where the number of people needing dialysis treatment is expected to increase.

RICK PERRY: GIVE SENIORS MORE SKIN IN THE GAME

Rick Perry, governor of Texas, had a diffuse menu of ideas for Medicare. He supported Paul Ryan's plan for premium support for seniors, and he favored South Carolina Republican Senator Jim DeMint's proposal to allow seniors to opt out of Medicare altogether and obtain private insurance. Such a plan is unrealistic because the cost of private insurance for seniors, who use more health care than any age group, would be prohibitive. Perry was inclined to means test Medicare, an idea favored by Republican Tom Coburn from Oklahoma and Joe Lieberman from Connecticut.

BUDDY ROEMER AND THE FIVE DOLLAR CONTRIBUTION FROM THE HEALTH CARE INDUSTRY

Americans heard very little about Buddy Roemer, a presidential candidate who joined the battle for the Republican nomination. He vowed not to take any money from special interests and had a one hundred dollar limit on campaign contributions.

"I'm free to lead because I take no corporate money," Roemer said. "I talk about things you need to hear." Total contributions from the health care industry were negligible, just five dollars, according to the Center for Responsive Politics.

A former four-time member of Congress and Governor of Louisiana, Roemer was not invited to participate in any of the televised Republican debates. "I can't even get into the debates," he said. Debate sponsors set the criteria for participating. To get into one debate, candidates had to raise at least half a million dollars in the previous ninety days, Roemer told the *PBS NewsHour.* "Is that the standard to elect our president?" he asked.

In another unusual move for a Republican, Roemer endorsed the Occupy Wall Street movement. "I believe they smell what's wrong with America," he said. "Wall Street and Washington, D.C. are connected at the pocketbook. America is bought and sold by the big companies and the special interests. . . . [President Obama] gets elected, and he says he wants change. But he takes all his money from these same corporations who don't want change." Roemer told supporters, "Wake up, America, they have stolen your government."

Roemer's prescription to sever the connection between Wall Street and Washington is clear and plainspoken. "The key issue in this country is to take the lobbyists out of the room . . . and let plain people in the room."

Candidates for president are like NASCAR drivers, as Roemer's campaign illustrated. They can join the race only if they have corporate sponsors. Once elected, Democrats and Republicans do the bidding for powerful corporate interests. They are work-for-hire presidents.

The story is not a new one. As Mark Twain quipped, "I think I can say, and say with pride, that we have some legislatures that bring higher prices than any in the world." The amount of money at stake is more than Twain could have imagined. Political campaigns have a price. A bidding war will keep prices headed north. This is why America no longer has presidents like Abraham Lincoln, who was honest, could not be bought, and took unpopular positions to move a country forward for the betterment of all.

Part V

SAVING MEDICARE

For more than thirty years, Republicans have proclaimed that competition will fix health care. Is it true? In chapter 14 we take a close look at competition in action to understand what it means for seniors when they choose among competing private health insurance plans and traditional Medicare. Curiously, proponents of health plan competition for seniors in the insurance market are silent when it comes to competition in the upstream wholesale market for hospital supplies and drugs, which could yield instant savings for Medicare worth billions of dollars. We wanted to know the reason for the silence, so we trace what happened when an advocate for price competition for prescription drugs tried to make the market really work for ordinary Americans and how he kicked a beehive.

In chapter 15 we highlight uncanny parallels between recent trends in the stock market and health care. Long-term investing in stocks has given way to short-term trading for quick profits, driving out mom-and-pop investors who invested in the market for the long haul. We couldn't help but notice that the same short-term mentality has gripped health care. Rather than making a long-term investment in Americans' health, the business-driven model in health care emphasizes short-term transactions, whether it is the seven-minute doctor visit or a prescription for a quick-fix pill. The business of health care makes money on the churn, the short-term trades. Value is out. Short-term profiteering is in.

Because companies are under tremendous pressure to make quarterly earnings targets to satisfy the new short-term mindset of the quick-money traders, we believe it is not enough for Medicare to change the financial incentives for how it pays providers to encourage them to take a longer-term view of patients' health. A far deeper fix is needed.

For that, we go upstream and look at the obligations of corporations in the business of health care and their duty in the marketplace. For-profit companies that make health care products such as drugs and devices, and those that provide health care in hospitals, hospices, home-care agencies, and long-term care, have a primary fiduciary duty to shareholders in their corporate statutes. They have no such primary duty to patients, their customers. We call for health care corporations to have a primary fiduciary duty to patients. While this recommendation is highly unlikely to be implemented, we offer it to show that a diagnosis of the root cause of Medicare's ills, and that of health care generally in the United States, stretches deep into the heart of the rules governing corporate behavior.

In the final chapter, we call for restoring Medicare to its rightful owners, the hardworking people who pay for it and seniors who rely on it. Restoration never happens quickly. It has taken a long time for Medicare to be molded by the nexus between Wall Street and Washington, and it will take a long time to loosen the ties. The chapter calls for reigniting Medicare's original purpose to provide health care security to older Americans and generations to come.

· *14* ·

Free Market or Market Failure?

*W*hen billionaire Donald Trump dallied with running as a candidate for the 2012 Republican presidential ticket, he proclaimed that the free market would solve the health care cost problem. Is he right?

"When I build a building, I let various building architects compete for the contract," Trump wrote. "Why? Because it sharpens their game, makes them bid competitively on price and encourages them to give me the best quality product possible. That's why Americans need more options when it comes to purchasing health care insurance."

Trump is not alone in saying that competition in a free market is the salve for the ills of health care. Stanford University economist John B. Taylor wrote that a key principle to guide Medicare should be "economic liberty and freedom to choose health care plans in a system that creates competing market conditions for insurance companies."

Americans have an abiding love for freedom. After all, freedom was the rallying cry when America was born from resistance to colonial oppressors in England. Americans want to be free to choose in the marketplace for cars, big-screen televisions, and smartphones.

The free market works well when new businesses can enter a market, compete, and offer more choice and high-quality products. Consumers drive out the bad actors, and good businesses thrive.

REALITY CHECK

When it comes to health care, does freedom to choose work? Let's take a look at how competition among private health insurance plans in

Medicare works in real life for America's seniors. To find out, take this test. Do a Google search on your computer for the word "Medicare" and see what appears.

When we did a search, the first entry that popped up was United-Healthcare supplemental Medicare insurance. Here's what it said: "Medicare doesn't pay for all of the costs of hospital and medical care. Consider AARP Medicare Supplement Plans, insured by UnitedHealthcare Insurance Company, to help with some of these costs."

The second search result was Humana, another corporate insurance giant, saying, "Get more benefits than original Medicare with a Medicare Advantage plan. Don't miss your chance to enroll!"

The third entry was a company that advertised free seminars for seniors every Monday morning in its suburban office-park location to help them understand their options. Its website is peppered with testimonials from satisfied customers who had pointed views about the array of Medicare choices. A customer wrote, "The volume and complexity of material pertaining to Medicare benefits make it very difficult for a lay person to even navigate the information terrain much less determine the option most suitable for his/her particular situation." Another senior opined, "Without your help, I would be lost." Yet another senior wrote with exasperation, "Medicare and the Part C and D . . . are so confusing, especially to seniors." A different user expressed relief, noting "the aggravation it would have taken me to do the research myself."

The fourth entry that came up in our Google search was the federal government's Medicare.gov website. When we typed in a zip code to find out the number of available Medicare insurance plan options, thirty prescription drug plans, six private health insurance plans with drug coverage, and four private health insurance plans without drug coverage were listed. The options are mind boggling even for veteran health policy wonks. In many communities across America—about one in four—seniors can choose from a bewildering array of at least thirty competing plans.

Most boomers and seniors say they don't understand Medicare, according to a survey conducted by the National Council on Aging and UnitedHealthcare. The majority said they did not know the purpose of the different parts of Medicare, and more than two-thirds did not understand Part C, the private health plan option. Faced with an overwhelming number of choices, seniors often make poor decisions, say researchers at Harvard Medical School.

Also consider that five million seniors over age sixty-five have Alzheimer's disease, and one-third of seniors over age eighty-five have trouble seeing even while wearing eyeglasses. Vision impairment impedes an informed choice.

Too many competing and confusing options creates opportunity for mischief. Americans learned from the mortgage meltdown that mortgage brokers and bankers often acted in their self-interest, giving loans to home buyers that made money for the brokers and the banks but wreaked havoc on families who could not afford them. In the same way, health insurance brokers can steer unsuspecting seniors to health insurance plans that give the broker the most lucrative commission even if the plan is not the best product for the customer.

Private health insurance companies that offer Medicare Advantage plans pay for the free seminars. The suburban location requires seniors to drive to attend them, which attracts those who are mobile and healthier. Private health plans prefer to "cherry-pick" healthier seniors to keep costs down.

Do seniors get advice that is best for them? The Medicare Rights Center, which advocates for the interests of seniors, says they are susceptible to misleading and aggressive marketing of private Medicare Advantage plans even after Congress passed legislation in 2008 to rein in egregious practices.

The center helped a seventy-eight-year-old South Carolina man whose insurance agent advised him to update his coverage. Although he was happy with his current Medicare plan, he switched based on the agent's recommendation. Soon, seven hundred dollars in copayments piled up because his doctors were not in the provider network, contrary to the information given by the agent. He could not find a local dentist that participated in the plan, so the promise of dental care was not true either. The South Carolina governor's office intervened on his behalf, as did the Medicare Rights Center. His prior Medicare plan enrolled him retroactively and covered most of the accumulated bills.

Americans want a fair market, not a free market. They want insurance that is simple and makes them feel secure. They don't want to worry about making the right choice or whether "premium support" or a "voucher" will cover the cost. Nor do they want to worry whether a private insurance company will deny payment for a treatment or test. Unwieldy competition has not produced this outcome. It breeds confusion and worry.

Test-driving an insurance plan isn't an option, nor is a trial run for surgery. Everyone pays for health insurance and treatment in advance. There is no money-back guarantee. If a treatment is effective, you pay. If it doesn't work, you pay. If a drug has terrible side effects, you can't return it. If a surgeon flubs a surgery, you'll probably still pay the copay. Reliable information about the quality of care and cost is sparse.

This is why the Nobel Prize–winning economist Kenneth Arrow wrote fifty years ago that a "laissez-faire solution for medicine is intolerable." Health care has unique features of uncertainty and risk, and he was right.

Competition and consumer choice in health care are not new ideas. During the Reagan administration, economists at the American Enterprise Institute and the Heritage Foundation promoted health care competition and choice. When applied to health insurance and health care services, the market doesn't work very well.

True devotees of free-market competition would be eager to instill competition in markets within the health care sector, where it would yield lower costs and improve the quality of products and services. Competition in the upstream wholesale market for hospital supplies and equipment, now the domain of group purchasing organizations, is an ideal example. Hospitals and other purchasers would save billions of dollars if they could buy products from a true Costco-like purchasing model. Curiously, competition in the wholesale market isn't promoted by advocates of competition. We wanted to understand why, so we ferreted out a true advocate of competition and learned the stark reality.

WHY REPUBLICANS DON'T LIKE *THIS* KIND OF COMPETITION

Governor Rick Perry, Republican governor of Texas and candidate for the Republican ticket in the 2012 presidential campaign, wrote in his book *Fed Up!*, "No issue is more critical to the defense of freedom and the American way of life than the preservation of our free-market health care system." Newt Gingrich penned the foreword.

In the Medicare prescription drug legislation that Gingrich championed, a free-market approach would have allowed the importation of prescription drugs from countries such as Canada, but the industry scuttled it. A drug such as Lipitor, which is used to treat cholesterol, is made in Ireland, imported to the United States, and shipped to Canada, but it cannot be imported back to America for sale at a lower price charged in Canada. During the legislative debate, Republican congressman Dan Burton, who wanted to legalize drug importation from Canada with safeguards, said, "That is unconscionable. . . . Here we are, going to spend billions and billions and billions and probably trillions of dollars on pharmaceutical products. . . . That's just not right."

That's what Michael Albano, mayor of Springfield, Massachusetts, thought too. To save his city and municipal workers money, he set up a prescription drug buying program in Canada for city employees, retirees, and their families. Health care spending was out of control, more than doubling in eight years, triggering layoffs of city teachers, firefighters, and policemen.

The city started the program with one-third of eligible employees, retirees, and dependents. Total costs for drugs dropped three million dollars.

Springfield is not a wealthy community, Albano said. Most children live at or below poverty and seniors cut their medicines in half so they last longer. Or they go without them.

"This was a good program that saved the city money," Albano said. "The average family saved a thousand dollars a year, and the average retiree saved four or five hundred dollars a year. We didn't even have a copay."

The city planned to include all ten thousand eligible people, but Albano began to feel the heat. He said he received a call from the U.S. Justice Department. "They threatened to indict me even though what I was doing was perfectly legal," he said to us. "The next day I held a press conference and invited everyone. I said, 'If you are going to indict me for getting lower prescription drug costs for my retirees, go ahead, make my day.'" That was the end of that, or so he thought.

Albano soon realized how deeply the system is stacked against good people who want to do the right thing. U.S. customs intercepted insulin for his son that had been mailed from a Canadian pharmacy. Albano had followed the law. He had a valid prescription. The drug purchase was for personal use, not resale. The amount was no more than a three-month supply.

Albano was spooked. He called the administrator of the Food and Drug Administration, Dr. Mark McClellan, to complain. Albano says he was told that it was just a coincidence. He didn't believe it. "They just wanted to make a point."

A Canadian pharmacist told *60 Minutes* that his pharmacy received letters from the big multinational companies threatening to cut off the pharmacy's drug supply if it continued to sell drugs to city workers in Springfield and elsewhere.

Albano left office when his term ended. When we asked him why he chose not to run for mayor for another term, he replied, "If I had stayed another two years, they would have tried to take me out in cuffs. I worked in the criminal justice system and know how those guys operate. They would have tried to find something to put me away. I'd just be getting out of jail now. I wonder what charge it would have been."

Albano was contacted by governments in Australia, Israel, and the United Kingdom that were eager to sell prescription drugs to his city workers at a competitive price. "They saw me going to Canada and said I should put out a call for proposals and let them respond. I was getting international play because they wanted to compete. It shows that if you open up the borders, prices in the U.S. would drop overnight."

When Mitt Romney became governor of Massachusetts, the state consolidated municipal and state employee health insurance. The intent was to lower the cost, at least theoretically. The state would not allow Springfield or any other city to buy cheaper drugs from Canada. Albano's plan was scrapped.

Albano concedes that he lost the battle. "We're never going to win. There's just too much money floating around. I've been in politics for a long time. I've never seen anything so powerful. There's just too much money that's corrupting the system. It's legalized corruption."

Rick Perry wrote in his book that "federal bureaucrats get to decide a lot of things for you." He doesn't tell the public the truth—that high-level government officials and the drug companies conspire against the interests of ordinary Americans. The system is rigged. This is the corruption that is pushing seniors and boomers, as well as the country, over the fiscal cliff.

THE ILLUSION OF CONSUMER CHOICE

Because we write about health care, people often tell us about their experiences in the health care system. A colleague of ours is a healthy fifty-year-old who went to his doctor and learned that his blood pressure was mildly elevated. The doctor immediately prescribed a drug to lower blood pressure.

High blood pressure is a serious medical condition. Doctors today say that uncontrolled hypertension was the cause of President Franklin Delano Roosevelt's massive brain hemorrhage on April 12, 1945, that led to his death. At that time, his doctors did not know the dangers of untreated hypertension. They thought Roosevelt was in excellent health and the cerebral hemorrhage "came out of the clear sky" when, in fact, his blood pressure had risen dramatically months earlier in November 1944 when he was reelected.

Our colleague's blood pressure was not nearly that high. It was mildly elevated yet required attention. He wanted to avoid taking blood pressure pills, if he could, and told his doctor that he wanted to change his diet and lose a few pounds before starting to take a pill every day. The doctor was not enthused and urged him to take the drug. The patient politely pushed back and left without a prescription.

He made modest changes in his diet and lost ten pounds. When he went back to the same doctor, his blood pressure was normal and the doctor told him he should keep doing whatever he was doing. Years later his blood pressure has remained normal and he is drug free, a small but important game changer. While lifestyle changes may not always be enough for some people, in his case, they were successful. He is empowered by this experience and is improving his health in other ways by changing the food he eats.

The health care system didn't support him when he sought to make a long-term investment in his health. No suggestions were made about foods that would help him rein in his blood pressure. In fact, the doctor discouraged him from taking ownership of his health.

Americans are given the illusion of choice rather than meaningful choice to invest in their health. Seniors can choose among multiple Medicare Part D prescription drugs plans. But they are rarely given the option to choose between a drug and alternatives that make it unnecessary.

Another friend of ours was taking medication for moderately high blood pressure that was well controlled. He began to feel short of breath while climbing stairs in his house. During a visit to a cardiologist, he had a series of tests that found blockages in three arteries. The doctor told him that he needed heart bypass surgery and scheduled it two weeks later.

He had the surgery and came home four days later. At first, he couldn't climb the four stairs to the front door of his house. Nor could he use his arms to turn over in bed or push himself out of bed because the pressure on his chest could tear open the sutures holding the sternum together. His wife rented a hospital bed for the basement, where he could enter through the garage. A week after he came home, he walked gingerly in his driveway. A few days later he ventured halfway down his street and turned around to go home because he was tired but wanted to talk about his experience. While he was in the hospital, tubes were placed in every opening of the body. "It's no time for modesty," he quipped.

Now he is back to work and goes camping with a local Boy Scout troop. He is happy to be alive. In the year after surgery, he lost twenty pounds and began walking two miles a day, down from three miles a day when he first began cardiac rehab.

Could he have been a candidate for a long-term investment in his health rather than major surgery that required sawing open his chest? We don't know the details of his medical condition. Nonetheless, we wondered if he could have reversed the disease without disturbing the inner sanctum of the human heart. Leading doctors say that heart bypass surgery is one of the most overused procedures in the United States. The night before his surgery, we read an extensive review of the history and evidence for the effectiveness of heart bypass surgery written by David Jones from the Department of the History of Science at Harvard. The risks of surgery are significant and include infection and cognitive impairment that affects 15 percent of people. The risk of death is always present.

In our book *The Treatment Trap*, we interviewed people who were told they needed heart bypass surgery or a heart transplant and were desperate to find an alternative that didn't involve surgery. They embarked on a formal, rigorous program to change what they ate, how they exercised, and how they lived their life. Benefits were quickly apparent. They regained the ability to walk and climb stairs without becoming short of breath. Chest pain subsided. Obvious improvements in their day-to-day life motivated them to continue.

They made the decision to invest in their health for the long term. Their cardiologists did not support their choice and, in most cases, scoffed at the idea that heart disease could be reversed. Nonetheless, they took the road less traveled and began a new chapter in their lives. It wasn't easy, but neither is major surgery. Their health insurance company paid for a lifestyle change program to help them regain their health.

Evidence demonstrates the efficacy of lifestyle changes. People with moderate to severe coronary heart disease who participated in a rigorous program to help them change their diet, increase physical activity, and reduce stress have reduced the blockages in their arteries, according to a study published in the *Journal of the American Medical Association*. The evidence revealed that many people can begin to reverse heart disease if they give their body the chance to heal itself.

In 2011 Medicare began to pay to help seniors change their lifestyle. To be eligible to participate in a Medicare-funded lifestyle change program, a senior must have had a heart attack in the past twelve months or have already had stable chest pain, heart bypass surgery, heart valve repair or replacement, a stent, or a heart transplant.

Most people will never hear about this alternative from their doctors. They will have to ferret it out on their own. Hospitals, doctors, and drug companies thrive on short-term transactions and starve when long-term investments create health.

The film *Forks Over Knives* is a reminder that even with the most advanced medical technology in the world, Americans are sicker than ever by nearly every measure. Heart disease, cancer, and stroke are the leading causes of death. Major surgeries are routine rather than the exception. As the country is on track to spend nearly three trillion dollars a year on health care, the American way is not making people healthier.

The film explores the idea that the best medicine may be the food that we eat. This is hardly new-age hype. Hippocrates advised more than two thousand years ago, "Let medicine be thy food and food be thy medicine." This philosophy underlies a program being tested by supermarket chain Whole Foods to bring a whole-health approach to a small group of its employees. The plan is to help team members make a long-term investment in their health, removing the need for a laundry list of prescription drugs.

HOW THE FREE MARKET IN HEALTH CARE ISN'T FREE

While we were writing this book, we were introduced to a former corporate vice president for employee benefits at a Fortune 10 company whose employees work around the country. We learned how an unfettered free market in health care can run amuck.

The company offered to pay for a second opinion when employees learned they had a serious medical condition. When employees were told they needed a heart or liver transplant, for example, the company offered to pay the cost of travel and a second opinion at first-rate places such as the Mayo Clinic.

Over the years, the company kept track of the impact of its second-opinion program. Forty percent of employees who were told they needed an organ transplant and received a second opinion learned they did not need it.

This was not a ploy by the company to cut costs. Take the case of an employee who was recommended for an organ transplant who went for a second opinion. He was told that he had cancer and was likely to die from it whether or not the transplant was performed. After he and his wife returned home, he died shortly thereafter from cancer as predicted. After his death, his wife received a phone call from the first hospital that wanted to do the transplant to ask when her husband wanted to schedule it.

Another employee was told he needed a heart transplant. When the company called the surgeon at a well-known institution to tell him that it was willing to pay for a second opinion, the surgeon said the patient shouldn't fly on a plane because of his medical condition. In fact, the employee has just traveled by plane to see the same surgeon and was more than delighted to obtain a second opinion, which revealed a small blockage successfully managed with a stent.

We have written about overtreatment in our book *The Treatment Trap*, but unnecessary transplants are one of the worst examples of overtreatment we have encountered. Because the supply of organs is limited, medically unnecessary transplants take life away from those who will die without one.

Hospitals are required to perform a minimum number of transplants each year to continue to qualify as a transplant center. A minimum volume ensures that the surgeon and team perform the procedure often enough and are competent. Transplants are financially lucrative. No one appears to hold transplant centers accountable for ensuring they are performing only medically necessary procedures.

Open markets can create wealth better than any other system. They were meant to be a rising tide that lifts all boats. But free markets need to be fair. Absent rules, monetary gain is created in the health care sector at the expense of others, sometimes in the most inhumane manner.

Unfettered competition in American health care, coupled with no limits on how much Medicare can spend each year, has caused an oversupply of hospitals, diagnostic imaging facilities, ambulatory surgery centers, and other facilities that are desperate for patients. In the Midwest, two hospitals that had collaborated began to see their revenue drop during the Great Recession. They ended their collaboration so they could ramp up their revenue. Each hospital replicated the services that the other hospital was providing. Hospital A built a cardiac center even though hospital B already had one. Meanwhile, hospital B built a new cancer center even though hospital A already had one.

Competition can work against the interests of patients. Consider Mr. Jones, who goes to a hospital with a medical condition that concerns him. The doctor diagnoses him and realizes that a competing hospital has a surgeon and team of nurses who are better equipped and trained to provide the best care for this patient. Yet the doctor is under pressure to meet productivity targets and to admit patients like Mr. Jones who have good health insurance. Will the doctor act in the best interest of the patient? Financial pressures too often trump what is right for the patient.

An oversupply of providers has not lowered prices in American health care. Nor has it led to better quality. It is easier for hospitals to spend money on advertising to create a perception of quality rather than create the reality of quality.

Medicare's open-ended entitlement, coupled with unfettered authority to build duplicative facilities and render unnecessary and potentially harmful treatment, have created the perfect storm of what a health care system should *not* do. Without red lights, American-style health care competition is driving America to the brink of financial disaster.

· 15 ·

Public Interest, Not Private Gain

$\mathcal{I}$t was a remarkably candid moment on Capitol Hill. The CEO of the New York Stock Exchange, Duncan Niederauer, told a hearing in the U.S. House of Representatives in June 2012 that the public is losing confidence in the stock market.

He explained how investors used to buy and hold stocks for the long term. The buy-and-hold strategy provided mom-and-pop investors a sense of ownership in big American icons such as Ford Motor Company and AT&T. Slow and steady returns would be the reward.

The buy-and-hold strategy has gone the way of the horse and buggy. Taking its place are high-frequency traders using computers and sophisticated software. Owned for mere seconds or hours, stocks are traded sometimes thousands of times a day. The numbers tell the story. The average time that stocks were held in 2012 was only three months compared with four years from 1926 to 1999.

The small investor cannot compete with the high-frequency trader whose eyes are glued to computer screens, nor with the machines and their software trolling for a few pennies in profit a share multiplied by thousands of shares.

"The citizenry has lost trust and confidence . . . in what used to be an investor's market [and] is now thought of as a trader's market," Niederauer said. The roller-coaster ride of volatility is driving away small, ordinary investors who can't stand the ride and know that the system is rigged. Lost in the trading mania is the time-honored notion of value. Value is out. Short-term profiteering is in.

WHAT HAPPENS ON WALL STREET
DOESN'T STAY ON WALL STREET

The market is unforgiving to companies in the business of health care that reel under constant pressure to show the money to their new masters, the high-frequency traders, rather than more patient mom-and-pop investors. Short-term profiteering provokes the frenetic pace that demands companies get drugs and devices to market faster than ever, whether or not they are ready for prime time in the human body. It demands higher "productivity" in hospitals, an ever-increasing pace for doctors and nurses that is impossible to maintain while also providing safe care.

The demanding pace spurs a lobbying onslaught to remove red lights in government regulation. Unbiased scientific studies are mere obstacles to company survival in a marketplace where losers take none. The market madness drives private equity firms to flip hospices in speculative pursuit of short-term gain.

The short-term mentality that grips companies trickles down to sick people in hospital beds and on exam tables in doctors' offices. Dialysis companies are goaded to administer more profit-making drugs into patients. It doesn't matter whether human life is cut short. What matters is whether financial targets are met in time for quarterly conference calls with investment analysts from hedge funds and private equity firms.

Niederauer is not alone in his assessment of the short-term fever that grips the stock market. Legendary investor Warren Buffet was joined by twenty-seven other stock-market gurus who issued a statement released by the Aspen Institute in 2009 titled "Overcoming Short-termism." Here is an excerpt:

> In recent years, boards, managers, shareholders with varying agendas, and regulators, all, to one degree or another, have allowed short-term considerations to overwhelm the desirable long-term growth and sustainable profit objectives of the corporation. We believe that short-term objectives have eroded faith in corporations continuing to be the foundation of the American free enterprise system, which has been, in turn, the foundation of our economy. Restoring that faith critically requires restoring a long-term focus for boards, managers, and most particularly, shareholders—if not voluntarily, then by appropriate regulation.

What does the switch from long-term investing to short-term profiteering have to do with Medicare? The changes in the stock market made us think about the short-term approach to *health care* in America compared with the long-term investment needed for good *health*. Here is an example of what we mean.

One day one of us met a woman in the grocery store who had an eye-catching pile of fresh fruit and vegetables stacked in her shopping cart. When asked about her healthy choices, she was eager to explain how she learned to eat healthy when she was a teenager. Forty years later at age fifty-nine, she is reaping the long-term investment she has made in her health. She uses little health care, takes no prescription drugs, goes to her doctor regularly for checkups, and is in remarkably good health. She will be eligible for Medicare in six years. If past performance is an indicator of future performance, she will be an infrequent flyer in her use of health care. She lamented the health status of her siblings, who consumed the all-American diet and are plagued with heart disease and diabetes and the requisite stream of visits to doctors and periodic hospitalizations.

Just as real wealth creation requires a long-term strategy, real health creation requires a long-term investment rather than short-term transactions. The seven-minute doctor visit lamented by doctors and patients alike is a classic case of the short-term transaction that occurs millions of times every day.

That said, there are extraordinary episodic interventions in American health care: the rescue of a teenager with asthma who sinks to the bottom of a swimming pool, unable to breathe, and is rescued; a fifty-eight-year-old who has a stroke while at a rest stop along Interstate 95 and receives perfect care at a nearby hospital and now lives a normal life; a member of Congress, Gabrielle Giffords from Arizona, who is shot in the head at point-blank range at a supermarket and survives.

This is America's health care that is brilliant and eminently satisfying to doctors, nurses, and patients. It is the culmination of years of study, practice, and fine-tuning so it becomes as perfect as humanly possible. This is the medicine that evokes awe and gratitude.

The American public has come to expect that other ills that afflict the human body respond to short-term fixes. Nothing can be further from the truth. Maintaining and improving health requires a long-term investment. Doctors and nurses can lend a hand, but all of us must make the investment ourselves, becoming good stewards of the body that will be inhabited for seventy or eighty years.

HOW MEDICARE PARTED WAYS
WITH A LONG-TERM INVESTOR

One of the early visionaries for what is now Medicare, President Harry Truman, understood the long-term investment that people need to make in their own health. In a speech at the Statler Hotel in Washington, DC, on May 1, 1948, he spoke about his hopes for a long-term investment strategy to improve the health of the American people:

> You know, [for] most of us, the reason we are not physically fit is because we are too lazy to take care of ourselves. We sit down and wait until this paunch comes on, and when we get bent over, then we try to correct it by heroic methods; and 9 times out of 10, if you go along and do what you ought to, in the first place, you wouldn't have that situation. What I want to do is to . . . keep people healthy, not to cure them after they get sick, or after they get beyond the point where they can be cured.

Today, no president would speak so openly and honestly. The media would spin the forthrightness as "blaming the victim" rather than a call to action for personal responsibility for one's own health.

Truman had two aims. First, he wanted people to know how to take care of their own health. He said, "I want to see the coming generation healthier and with a better outlook on life than we had when we were growing up. In order to do that, you have got to educate people. You have got to educate young people. You have got to tell them how to take care of themselves."

Then Truman talked about health care. "You have got to have a medical profession and a hospital organization program that can meet that situation, and that the people can afford to pay for," he said. Together, these steps would help "make the greatest machine—the machine that God made—work as he intended it."

Medicare did not include the first part of Truman's vision. In fact, it was totally ignored. That's because Medicare's chief architects included the incipient medical-industrial complex: the American Medical Association, hospitals, and Blue Cross and Blue Shield. No powerful interest groups lobbied for a long-term investment in the public's health in the halls of Congress and the corridors of the White House.

The same is true today. The health care reform law, the Patient Protection and Affordable Care Act, provided seniors with new Medicare benefits. Seniors can have mammograms and colonoscopies without paying any copays. Prevention is defined as short-term, episodic interventions that put more money in the pockets of the health care industry. It isn't defined as helping people take charge of their own health.

Today, with 18 percent of the country's income spent on health care, a long-term investment in health is a do-it-yourself proposition. If you want to learn how to live a healthier life, the health care system is not the place to go.

TRADERS OR INVESTORS?

If the Aspen Institute statement by Warren Buffet and fellow stock-market gurus was changed to apply to health care, the message is an eye-opener. Here is what it would say:

> In recent years, boards, managers, shareholders with varying agendas, and regulators, all, to one degree or another, have allowed short-term considerations to overwhelm the desirable long-term health of Americans. We believe that short-term objectives have eroded faith in the health care system as currently designed. Restoring that faith critically requires restoring a long-term focus for boards, managers, and most particularly, shareholders—if not voluntarily, then by appropriate regulation.

In their joint statement, the gurus identify three consequences of short-term trading in the stock market. Each one can be applied to health care.

Frequent Trading Increases Costs

The financial gurus say, "High rates of portfolio turnover harm ultimate investors' returns, since the costs associated with frequent trading can significantly erode gains."

The same is true in American-style, revolving-door medicine. With the scarcity of primary-care doctors and geriatricians, boomers and seniors typically go to multiple doctors who don't coordinate their recommendations or treatment. The cardiologist looks at the heart. The rheumatologist looks at the joints. The dermatologist looks at the skin. No one examines the whole person.

A physician colleague with a number of medical issues told us about his experience getting his blood pressure under control. Three visits to his primary-care doctor over three months were needed. During the first office visit, the doctor was late because of an emergency with another patient and had only a few minutes to talk. At a second appointment that lasted about ten minutes, the situation was still not resolved. In a third visit, a nurse practitioner listened and made a few tweaks. Now our colleague is able to manage his blood pressure. The health insurance company and the patient paid for three office visits rather than one productive visit. More frequent, costly transactions impede gains that can be made with a more timely and effective intervention.

New York Stock Exchange CEO Duncan Niederauer said during his congressional testimony, "We convinced ourselves along the way that speed is synonymous with quality and in some cases it might be. In other cases, it clearly isn't." The same is true in health care. Speed makes all the difference in emergencies. In other cases, speed impedes quality.

Medicare officials are heroically trying to curb short-term practices and create conditions for long-term investments in health by helping doctors establish medical homes designed to support a team-based approach to coordinating care. For the foreseeable future, there will be too few medical homes to allow a broad-based impact. Nonetheless, they are a step in the right direction. Medicare officials are also trying to pay hospitals and doctors differently to encourage longer-term investments and discourage so many short-term trades. In the meantime, the revolving door swings fast and furious, increasing costs and, at times, causing more harm than good.

Short-Term Thinking Leads to Market Failure

The stock-market gurus say, "Fund managers with a primary focus on short-term trading gains have little reason to care about long-term performance and are unlikely to promote corporate policies and governance policies that are beneficial and sustainable in the long-term. The consequences of high-risk strategies designed exclusively to produce high returns in the short-run are evident in recent market failures."

In health care, defective metal-on-metal hip implants are an example of a high-risk corporate strategy that produced high returns in the short-run but failed to account for long-term performance. The market failure occurred when tens of thousands of people were harmed before the product was removed from the market.

Short-Term Actions Can Harm the Real Owners

The stock-market gurus say, "The focus of some short-term investors on quarterly earnings and other short-term metrics can harm the interests of shareholders seeking long-term growth and sustainable earnings."

For-profit hospital company HCA focused on short-term quarterly results and increased the number of cardiac procedures performed even when many of them were medically unnecessary and put people at risk. Patients who were looking for long-term health were harmed by the company's incessant short-term focus on quarterly earnings.

Duncan Niederauer told Congress, "The public has never been more disconnected. . . . The citizenry has lost trust and confidence" in the stock market. Meanwhile, the public has never been more unhappy about its health care. In a hyperactive world with pressure to "make the numbers," trust and confidence are impossible to build and sustain whether in financial markets or health care.

FROM STEWARDSHIP TO SALESMANSHIP

The legendary founder of Vanguard Funds and the father of the index fund, John Bogle, spoke about equity markets in a speech at Columbia University School of Business in 2009, a few months after the financial meltdown that triggered the Great Recession. His diagnosis of the meltdown's cause was the failure of corporations to fulfill their fiduciary duty to their shareholders. Short-term profiteering took precedence over duty to the investors they are obliged by law to serve. Here is what Bogle said, in part:

> As a group, we veered off course almost 180 degrees from steward-ship to salesmanship, in which our focus turned away from prudent

management and toward product marketing. We moved from a focus on long-term investment to a focus on short-term speculation. The driving dream of our adviser/agents was to gather ever-increasing assets under management, better to build their advisory fees and profits, even as these policies came at the direct expense of the investor/principles whom, under traditional standards of trusteeship and fiduciary duty, they were duty-bound to serve.

This same reasoning explains how the health care industry has veered off course into short-term profiteering at the expense of long-term investments in health. Here we adapt Bogle's words to health care, and the parallel implications are stunning:

As a group, we veered off course almost 180 degrees from stewardship to salesmanship, in which our focus turned away from prudent management of a patient's health to product marketing. We moved from a focus on long-term investment in our patients' health to a focus on short-term office visits, tests, procedures, drugs, and devices. The driving dream of the executives has been to build their fees and profits, even as those policies came at the direct expense of the patients whom, under traditional standards of ethical duty, they were duty-bound to serve.

Bogle is no shrinking capitalist. Yet he observes how many money managers on Wall Street strayed from the fiduciary principle by:

- Creating exotic and untested "products" that have far more ephemeral marketing appeal than investment integrity
- Managing assets for enormously high fees
- Spending enormous amounts on advertising to bring in new investors using money obtained from existing fund shareholders

The health care industry has strayed, too, from service to the patient by:

- Creating exotic and insufficiently tested drugs, devices, and surgical procedures that have far more ephemeral marketing appeal than medical purpose and integrity
- Managing health care assets and charging enormously high prices for hospital services, equipment, and drugs

- Spending enormous amounts on advertising to bring in new patients using money from existing patients

WHEN THERE IS NO DUTY TO THE PATIENT

The purpose of a corporation, according to the laws that establish them, is to make money for its shareholders. Boards of directors have a legal duty, a fiduciary duty, to owners to make money. Board members can be sued individually if they fail to carry out that duty. Bogle pointedly states that because many corporations have failed to carry out their duty faithfully, the very foundations of capitalism itself have been shaken, causing massive upheaval in society as millions of people lost their jobs and homes in the Great Recession.

Similarly, the laws governing investor-owned corporations that make health care products such as drugs and devices, and provide hospital and hospice care, require fiduciary duty to shareholders. There is no primary fiduciary duty to patients.

If banks and investment firms disrupted society by failing to fulfill their legal duty to their shareholders, how much disruption do health care corporations cause when they have no fiduciary duty to the sick embedded in the laws that create them?

To begin to answer this question, we look to Justice Harlan Fiske Stone, who gave an address at the University of Michigan law school during the Great Depression in the 1930s. Like Bogle, Justice Stone chastised corporations and their boards for their failure to live up to their duty to their shareholders. Here is what Stone said:

> I venture to assert that when the history of the financial era which has just drawn to a close comes to be written, most of its mistakes and its major faults will be ascribed to the failure to observe the fiduciary principle, the precept as old as holy writ, that "a man cannot serve two masters." No thinking man can believe that an economy built upon a business foundation can permanently endure without some loyalty to that principle. The separation of ownership from management, the development of the corporate structure so as to vest in small groups control over the resources of great numbers of small and uninformed investors, make imperative a

fresh and active devotion to that principle if the modern world of business is to perform its proper function.

Yet those who serve nominally as trustees, but relieved, by clever legal devices, from the obligation to protect those whose interests they purport to represent, corporate officers and directors who award to themselves huge bonuses from corporate funds without the assent or even the knowledge of their stockholders . . . suggest how far we have ignored the necessary implications of that principle. The loss and suffering inflicted on individuals, the harm done to a social order founded upon business and dependent upon its integrity, are incalculable.

Here is what happens when health care companies, whose business is the care of the patient, have no legal duty to that patient in the laws governing their operations. We adapt Justice Stone's statement to give the answer:

We venture to assert that when the history of health care in America is written, most of its mistakes and its major faults will be ascribed to the failure to observe the fiduciary principle, the precept as old as holy writ, that "a person cannot serve two masters." No thinking person can believe that a health care system built upon a business foundation can permanently endure without some loyalty to the patient. The separation of the real owners, the patients, from management, and the development of increasingly hierarchical health care organizations that vest in small groups control over the resources meant to be used for great numbers of small and uninformed patients, make imperative a fresh and active devotion to the principle of fiduciary duty to the patient if modern health care is to perform its proper function.

Yet those who serve nominally as trustees are relieved, by clever legal devices, from the obligation to protect the interests of the patients they ultimately serve. Corporate officers and directors award to themselves huge bonuses from corporate funds while patients who need their health restored may have modest means. Institutions consider only last, if at all, the interests of the patients for whom the entire health care enterprise was established. We have ignored the principle of fiduciary duty, which requires loyalty to the patient. The loss and suffering inflicted on individuals, the harm done to a social order founded upon business and dependent upon its integrity, are incalculable.

The most fundamental challenge facing Medicare and all of health care in America is that it serves two masters: private gain and the patient. Private gain driven by greed—the same greed that caused the Great Depression and the Great Recession—is the tragic flaw that will cause the meltdown of Medicare. If Medicare collapses, the entire economy will be under such stress that it, too, will stumble.

Federal regulations finalized during the Obama administration made fiduciary duty to the patient an even more distant reality. New entities called accountable care organizations (ACOs) were authorized in the Patient Protection and Affordable Care Act. Their purpose is to coordinate care among hospitals, doctors, and other providers and be financially rewarded for doing so. Regulations require them to have a fiduciary duty to the ACO and to act consistent with that duty. Medicare officials did not require primary fiduciary duty to the patient.

What does this mean for you? If you go to a doctor who is employed by a hospital that is part of an accountable care organization, and if he or she feels that you would be best served by a doctor in another competing organization, the doctor has a duty to you as a patient, but the organization where the doctor works does not.

Twenty public-interest groups and individuals, including Health-Watch USA, Mothers Against Medical Error, Cautious Patient Foundation, Citizen Advocacy Center, Empowered Patient Coalition, New Hampshire Patient Voices, and the Connecticut Center for Patient Safety, were among those that wrote to Medicare officials calling for a change to the regulation governing ACOs. They recommended that primary duty should be to the patient. Medicare officials did not respond.

ESTABLISH CORPORATE FIDUCIARY DUTY TO THE PATIENT

As Medicare approaches its fiftieth anniversary, it is timely to consider whether corporations, whose businesses have a direct impact on the health and well-being of seniors and all Americans, should be required by law to have a fiduciary duty to the patient.

A former corporate lawyer, Robert Hinckley, who left practice to inform the public how laws governing corporations place private gain above the public interests, wrote, "Corporate law . . . casts ethical and social concerns as irrelevant, or as stumbling blocks to the corporation's fundamental mandate. The law governing corporations builds in active disregard for the harm to all interests other than those of shareholders."

Yet corporate directors are personally liable for false and misleading statements in the prospectuses used to sell securities.

> If a corporate prospectus contains a material falsehood and investors suffer damage as a result, investors can sue each director personally to recover the damage. . . . Similarly, everyone who works on the prospectus knows that directors' personal wealth is at stake, so they too take great care with accuracy.

What if corporate directors were held personally responsible for preventable harm to seniors and all Americans? They would not let companies sell drugs and devices that have known flaws, nor enroll patients in hospice who are not dying, administer excess drugs to kidney dialysis patients that increase the chance of death, nor perform surgeries on patients that cause more harm than good. Accountability will be hardwired into the system.

Turning this idea into practice may be impossible. The limited liability of corporations has become ingrained in the psyche of business. But the first step to cure an illness, especially a terminal one, is the correct diagnosis, even if few want to hear it. Ensuring loyalty to the patient is the most fundamental challenge to Medicare and Americans of all ages.

Many doctors and nurses will support a requirement that the governing boards of the organizations where they work have a duty to the patients just as they do. They don't want to go to work every day in places that lack a primary duty to the patient as a first and foremost principle. The conflict and moral distress that ensue are immeasurable. They are asked to serve two masters and cannot do so faithfully. It is unethical to place the magnitude of the conflict of interest built into the entire health care system on the consciences of people on the front lines, at the sharp end, where it ultimately matters.

The Nobel laureate and economist Kenneth Arrow once wrote, "Virtually every commercial transaction has within itself an element of trust." Health care is more than a mere commercial exchange. It is a matter of life and death. A person places his or her trust not only in doctors and nurses but in the organization that renders the service. Loyalty to the patient should be its primary duty.

As it stands today, irreconcilable differences exist today between the demands of the publicly held corporation and duty to the patient. The only way to resolve these differences may be a divorce of health care from the traditional laws governing corporations, or a revision of those laws.

The proposal is radical, but it goes to the heart of filling the vacuum in accountability that exists in health care today. Responsibility for safe products and services belongs to their producers. While this may be an anathema to corporations, think for a moment how individuals are legally accountable for keeping their sidewalks clear of snow in the winter. Doing so helps a community function for the common good, for children walking to school or their parents walking to the bus or subway to go to work. Why should corporations skirt accountability for safety on a much larger scale affecting millions of people? By placing responsibility for safety and the cost of mitigating harm in the hands of companies, the incentives for safe care will change overnight.

Will corporate profits decline? Yes, they will decline because the costs of harm that are presently socialized, borne by patients, and spread among society will be internalized by the respective companies.

If this is troubling to you as an investor, think about this truth. If you own stocks in health care companies, realize that laws governing the establishment of the corporation specify that the firms that make the drugs you consume and devices that may be implanted in your body have no accountability to you. Corporate officers have a duty to their shareholders, not you. This truth should give you pause to ponder the mismatch between the legal framework of companies in the business of health care and your desire for safe, reliable medical care when it really counts.

· *16* ·

Recycle Medicare Waste:
Five Steps to Save Lots of Money

*A*fter the 2012 presidential election, a *New York Times* editorial reported that President Obama's 2013 budget proposed to cut $340 billion over ten years from Medicare by raising premiums on high-income beneficiaries, cutting payments to health care providers, and requiring drug companies to pay rebates to Medicare. The editors opined that besides these steps, "there are very limited options for further reducing Medicare . . . spending."

In fact, there are lots of ways for Medicare to save money. The place to look is the estimated $170 billion in annual Medicare waste reported by the Institute of Medicine. Policy makers and the media need to know where it goes, who is getting it, and what they are doing with it. Americans should be asking, "Why are we paying for all that waste?"

With all the waste in Medicare, the debate should not be about raising the eligibility age for Medicare, or increasing premiums. Seniors' entitlement to Medicare is not the problem to be fixed, nor the place where cuts should be made. This is the wrong conversation.

Companies that make money from the waste have a sense of entitlement to that money. *This* is the entitlement that needs to be cut.

Throughout this book, we have pulled back the curtain to reveal the waste. Here is a starter list to tackle it. It includes sixteen billion dollars' worth of appetizers on a larger menu of possible cuts. Even better, they tackle the underlying drivers of Medicare spending. Raising premiums and the eligibility age perpetuates the waste and doesn't cut costs.

Democrats and Republicans have put on the table the option of raising the Medicare eligibility age from sixty-five to sixty-seven. This will save $148 billion from 2012 to 2021, or about $15 billion a year, according to the Congressional Budget Office.

There are far better ways to save $15 billion a year. If the public could vote on options to save money, they would vote for these:

1. CREATE A COSTCO FOR HOSPITAL SUPPLIES AND EQUIPMENT: SAVE $5 BILLION A YEAR

The two-hundred-billion-dollar market for hospital supplies and equipment is riddled with waste. It accounts for nearly 8 percent of total health care spending in the United States. The market should operate like Costco and provide the most favorable deal to customers, in this case hospitals, ambulatory surgery centers, and other health care facilities that purchase everything from alcohol dispensers to oxygen tanks, infusion pumps, and CT scanners.

Congress needs to repeal the exemption from the federal anti-kickback law that benefits the few group-purchasing organizations that dominate the market. These organizations have the incentive to sell the most expensive products, at the highest possible volume, to health care facilities. This is why many hospitals around the country have expired and unused supplies in their inventory, as we revealed in chapter 11.

Proponents of competition and choice would be wise to direct their attention to fixing this market with price transparency and competition. Hospitals would save money, and they could better absorb reduced Medicare payments.

Savings of just 10 percent in this market would total twenty billion dollars a year. Medicare's share of the savings could be as much as five billion dollars annually because it accounts for about one-quarter of total health care spending. Even more savings can be gained from improving efficiency in this market.

Opposition from product manufacturers will be swift and fierce. But the option should be on the table so policymakers, the media, and the public know that there are ways to put Medicare on a sustainable financial footing without asking seniors and taxpayers to pay more.

2. CUT IMPROPER PAYMENTS TO HOSPITALS AND DOCTORS: SAVE $4.8 BILLION A YEAR

Medicare officials estimate that the program pays forty-eight billion dollars a year in improper payments. While some of these payments occur because of billing mistakes, the improper payments that everyone should be worried about are those made to hospitals and doctors for unnecessary heart surgeries, angioplasties, stents, and cardiac defibrillators, to name a few overused procedures.

Seniors receive no benefit, and worse, they are exposed to unnecessary risk and possible harm. The prevailing culture—"They harm you and they bill you for it"—needs to stop.

Medicare officials are trying hard to pare back improper payments. They receive a tsunami-like push back from hospitals and doctors who frame the issue as cutting patient access to care. If the public only knew the extent of improper payments and the harm they can cause, its voice could help fight an industry that believes it is entitled to the public's money when it bills for medically inappropriate services.

If just 10 percent of Medicare's improper payments can be stopped, Medicare would save nearly five billion dollars a year.

3. CUT MEDICARE PAYMENTS TO HOSPITALS FOR ROUTINE DOCTOR VISITS: SAVE $1 BILLION A YEAR

In 2011 Medicare paid about 80 percent more for a fifteen-minute office visit in a hospital outpatient department than if the same visit took place in a doctor's private office. Seniors pay higher copayments too.

As physicians sell their practices to hospitals in record numbers, more routine visits are occurring in hospital outpatient departments. Medicare Part B costs will increase dramatically and seniors will bear more of a burden without receiving any benefit.

The Medicare Payment Advisory Commission recommends that Congress authorize Medicare to pay the same amount no matter where the service is provided. This recommendation should be implemented. Medicare would save one billion dollars a year.

4. TACKLE MEDICARE FRAUD
AS IF IT MATTERED: SAVE $6 BILLION A YEAR

The Federal Bureau of Investigation estimates that up to 10 percent of health care spending is lost to fraud. In the case of Medicare, fraud consumes nearly $60 billion a year.

There is usually a lot more said than done about reducing Medicare fraud. Still, reducing fraud is not being widely discussed as a large part of the solution. Democrats and Republicans are putting Medicare eligibility on the chopping block to save fifteen billion dollars a year. Yet a similar push for curbing sixty billion in Medicare fraud is rarely whispered.

Cutting fraud by a mere 10 percent yields $5.6 billion in Medicare savings. Much more savings should be expected in subsequent years.

5. CAP MEDICARE SPENDING GROWTH

Both Democratic and Republican proposals to reform Medicare would cap how much Medicare spending can increase each year. A cap should be implemented. It will send a signal that Medicare should be no different than any other enterprise that has a budget and spending limits. Every family has a budget. Every business has a budget. Every Girl Scout troop has a budget. So does every place of worship. Medicare needs a budget too.

With a budget, the conversation in Washington will change from how to control Medicare spending to how the public's money can be used wisely to achieve the best health for millions of seniors.

Special interests will stir up a media frenzy to scare seniors. They will accuse the government of rationing care. After reading this book, you will have a better idea of what they are really up to.

Massachusetts is the first state to pull the emergency brake on health care spending. A law enacted in August 2012 aims to limit health care spending increases in line with the growth in the state's economy.

The state's actions are noteworthy because health care is big business in Massachusetts. Stakeholders realize that the state's signature achievement of nearly universal health insurance coverage will erode if health care becomes even more expensive than it is now. Health insurance will become like Swiss cheese with more holes than cheese.

Although the Massachusetts legislature and governor had the political will to vote to slow the growth of total health care spending, the law is aspirational. Nothing in the law stops the state's health care industry from trying to circumvent the caps. The law will be effective only with the political will to enforce it.

If Medicare spending is not put on a sustainable path, forces outside the control of the White House and Capitol Hill will drive cuts. A spike in interest rates charged to the federal government to borrow money, or a pullback by a major lender to the U.S. Treasury, could force cuts. They will be made with a meat cleaver rather than a scalpel that surgically removes the fat and leaves the lean.

With targeted cuts in waste, fraud, and abuse, no care needs to be rationed and no older Americans need to worry. Their hard-earned money will be used as it was intended, not to prop up an industry that relies on the blind generosity of the public.

Notes

CHAPTER 1

9 "Medicare is a huge program . . ." Congressional Budget Office, "The Budget and Economic Outlook," January 2012, 49, http://www.cbo.gov/sites/default/files/cbofiles/attachments/01-31-2012_Outlook.pdf, accessed July 1, 2012.

10 "This amount is more than . . . " CIA World Factbook, https://www.cia.gov/library/publications/the-world-factbook/fields/2195.html?countryName=New%20Zealand&countryCode=nz&regionCode=au&, accessed May 20, 2012.

10 "This is equivalent to adding more than the entire current populations . . ." CIA World Factbook, https://www.cia.gov/library/publications/the-world-factbook/rankorder/rawdata_2119.txt, accessed June 16, 2012.

10 "Sixty thousand dollars . . ." University of Michigan Office of the Registrar, "Tuition & Fees—Ann Arbor," http://www.ro.umich.edu/tuition/, accessed September 10, 2012; Harvard College Office of Admissions, "Cost of Attendance for 2012–2013," http://www.admissions.college.harvard.edu/financial_aid/cost.html, accessed September 10, 2012.

10 "Many Americans will work . . ." U.S. Census Bureau, "Quick Facts," http://quickfacts.census.gov/qfd/states/00000.html, accessed September 10, 2012. Median household income for 2006–2010 was $51,914.

11 "When he retired in 2011 . . ." C. Eugene Steuerle and Stephanie Rennane, "Social Security and Medicare Taxes and Benefits over a Lifetime," Urban Institute, June 2011, http://www.urban.org/UploadedPDF/social-security-medicare-benefits-over-lifetime.pdf, accessed September 2, 2012.

12 "Medicare payroll tax revenue . . ." "2012 Annual Report of the Boards of Trustees of the Federal Hospital Insurance and Federal Supplementary

Medical Insurance Trust Fund," April 23, 2012, 210, http://www.cms
.gov/Research-Statistics-Data-and-Systems/Statistics-Trends-and-Reports/
ReportsTrustFunds/Downloads/TR2012.pdf, accessed October 31, 2012.

12 "Not all of them make it to the Fortune . . ." "Fortune 500," *CNNMoney*,
2012, http://money.cnn.com/magazines/fortune/fortune500/2012/full_list/,
accessed June 29, 2012.

13 "Seventy-six percent of Fortune 50 . . ." PricewaterhouseCoopers, "Impact of Health Reform on Business Sectors," http://www.pwc.com/us/en/
health-industries/topics/health-reform.jhtml, accessed October 31, 2012.

13 "The notion that somehow we can . . ." President Barack Obama, Press Briefing, June 23, 2009, http://www.nytimes.com/2009/06/23/us/politics/23text
-obama.html?pagewanted=all&_moc.semityn.www, accessed June 30, 2010.

13 "Meanwhile, Limbaugh said . . ." Rush Limbaugh, "The Truth about
Medicare," transcript, May 25, 2011, http://www.rushlimbaugh.com/
daily/2011/05/25/the_truth_about_medicare, accessed October 31, 2012.

14 "For the foreseeable future . . ." The Congressional Budget Office projects
under its extended baseline scenario that Medicare will account for 6 percent
of GDP in 2035. See "CBO's 2011 Long-Term Budget Outlook," June
2011, 45–46, http://cbo.gov/sites/default/files/cbofiles/attachments/06-21
-Long-Term_Budget_Outlook.pdf, accessed June 20, 2012.

14 "In 2010, only . . ." American Geriatrics Society, "The Demand for Geri-
atric Care and the Evident Shortage of Geriatrics Healthcare Providers," June
2012, http://www.americangeriatrics.org/files/documents/Adv_Resources/
PayReform_fact5.pdf, accessed September 1, 2012.

14 "The median salary . . ." American Geriatrics Society, "Loan Debt and Salary Statistics for Geriatrics Healthcare Providers," June 2012, http://www
.americangeriatrics.org/files/documents/Adv_Resources/PayReform_fact4
.pdf, accessed September 1, 2012.

15 "Medicare will have only enough . . ." "2012 Annual Report of the Board
of Trustees of the Federal Hospital Insurance and Federal Supplementary
Medical Insurance Trust Fund," April 23, 2012, 31, http://www.cms.gov/
Research-Statistics-Data-and-Systems/Statistics-Trends-and-Reports/Reports
TrustFunds/Downloads/TR2012.pdf, accessed August 10, 2012.

15 "Beneficiary access to health care . . ." Ibid., 28.

15 "The first warning . . ." Michael O. Leavitt, "Letter from the Secretary of
the Department of Health and Human Services to the Speaker of the House
of Representatives and the President of the Senate," http://www.hhs.gov/
asl/medicarefundingwarningtransmittal.html, accessed July 8, 2012.

15 "More warnings have been . . ." "2009 Annual Report of the Boards of
Trustees of the Federal Hospital Insurance and Federal Supplementary Medi-
cal Insurance Trust Funds," May 12, 2009, 3, http://www.cms.gov/Reports
TrustFunds/downloads/tr2009.pdf, accessed September 12, 2012.

15 "In 2012 Secretary of the . . ." "A Summary of the 2012 Annual Reports, Social Security and Medicare Boards of Trustees," http://www.ssa.gov/oact/TRSUM/index.html, accessed July 8, 2012.

CHAPTER 2

17 "Comedian and social commentator . . ." "George Carlin on American Owners and Education," *YouTube,* http://www.youtube.com/watch?v=4jQT7_rVxAE, accessed June 17, 2012.

17 "During the 2000 presidential . . ." "Excerpts from Prepared Remarks by Bush and Gore," *New York Times,* May 16, 2000, http://www.nytimes.com/2000/05/16/us/excerpts-from-prepared-remarks-by-bush-and-gore.html?pagewanted=all&src=pm, accessed June 29, 2012.

17 "Less than four . . ." New York Stock Exchange, "Dow Jones Industrial Average (DJIA) History," http://www.nyse.tv/dow-jones-industrial-average-history-djia.htm, accessed July 15, 2012.

17 "Every month . . ." U.S. Social Security Administration, "Annual Statistics Supplement, 2010," table 5.A4, http://www.ssa.gov/policy/docs/statcomps/supplement/2010/5a.html#table5.a4, accessed August 30, 2012.

17 "During a presidential debate . . ." "Al Gore on Social Security," *On the Issues,* October 3, 2000, http://www.ontheissues.org/text/Al_Gore_Social_Security.htm, accessed July 3, 2012.

18 "This is asset accumulation . . ." "George Bush on Social Security," http://www.youtube.com/watch?v=dVy3VRLU2Js, accessed June 12, 2012.

18 "By October 2006 . . ." "Stock Market History," *Money-Zine,* http://www.money-zine.com/Investing/Stocks/Stock-Market-History/, accessed May 26, 2012.

19 "When all the out-of-pocket costs . . ." "2011 Annual Report of the Boards of Trustees of the Federal Hospital Insurance and Federal Supplementary Medical Insurance Trust Fund," May 13, 2011, 103, http://www.cms.gov/ReportsTrustFunds/downloads/tr2011.pdf, accessed December 28, 2011. See also Alison M. Shelton, "The Impact of Medicare Premiums on Social Security Beneficiaries," Congressional Research Service, Prepared for the Senate Committee on Aging, January 27, 2010, http://aging.senate.gov/crs/ss20.pdf, accessed January 2, 2012.

CHAPTER 3

21 "If Medicare spending continues . . ." Gooloo S. Wunderlich, "Improving Health Care Cost Projections for the Medicare Population: Summary of a Workshop" (Washington, DC: National Academies Press, 2010), http://www.nap.edu/catalog.php?record_id=12985, accessed July 17, 2012. See also Congressional Budget Office, "The Long-Term Outlook for Health Care Spending," November 2007, appendix D, p. 35, http://www.cbo.gov/sites/default/files/cbofiles/ftpdocs/87xx/doc8758/11-13-lt-health.pdf, accessed August 5, 2012.

22 "The 2012 Medicare trustees . . ." John N. Friedman, "Appendix A: Predicting Medicare Cost Growth," in Wunderlich, "Improving Health Care Cost Projections," 83–106, http://http://www.nap.edu/openbook.php?record_id=12985&page=83, accessed July 14, 2012.

24 "Together, these three . . ." Congressional Budget Office, "Letter from Douglas Elmendorf to John Boehner," July 24, 2012, 18, http://www.cbo.gov/sites/default/files/cbofiles/attachments/43471-hr6079.pdf, accessed December 3, 2012.

24 "The total reduction in payments . . ." Ibid., 14.

24 "Total reductions will be . . ." Ibid. Note that the $716 billion in Medicare spending cuts are calculated as follows: Part A (hospital insurance) and Part B (medical insurance) would total $517 billion and $247 billion, respectively. Those cuts would be partially offset by a $48 billion increase in net spending for Part D.

25 "If you wait . . ." Jennifer Haberkorn, "Ryan, Wyden Back a New Medicare Option," *Politico*, December 14, 2011, http://paulryan.house.gov/News/DocumentPrint.aspx?DocumentID=272601, accessed July 1, 2012.

25 "I'm against Obamacare . . ." "Meet the Press Transcript for May 15, 2011," *MSNBC.com*, May 15, 2011, http://www.msnbc.msn.com/id/43022759/ns/meet_the_press-transcripts/t/meet-press-transcript-may/#.Tws0m_lO_Lk, accessed July 1, 2012.

26 "I simply believe . . ." Haberkorn, "Ryan, Wyden Back a New Medicare Option."

26 "Robert Pear wrote in the . . ." Robert Pear, "Despite Democrats' Warnings, Private Medicare Plans Find Success," *New York Times*, August 26, 2012, 14.

26 "Seniors who have . . ." Kaiser Family Foundation, *Medicare Chartbook*, 4th ed., 2010, section 7, "Out-of-Pocket Spending," http://www.kff.org/medicare/upload/8103.pdf, accessed July 14, 2012.

27 "The Congressional Budget Office predicts . . ." Congressional Budget Office, "Comparison of Projected Enrollment in Medicare Advantage Plans," 2.

30 "My view is that . . ." Ricardo Alonso-Zaldivar, "House Republicans to Repeal Health Care Law's Independent Payment Advisory Board," *Huffington Post*, March 20, 2012, http://www.huffingtonpost.com/2012/03/20/gop-health-care-repeal-independent-payment-advisory-board_n_1367629.html, accessed July 17, 2012.

30 "Congress has always . . ." Pete Stark, "Statement of Pete Stark, Ranking Member, Ways and Means Subcommittee on Health, Hearing on the Independent Payment Advisory Board," press release, March 6, 2012, http://stark.house .gov/index.php?option=com_content&view=article&id=2374:press-release -stark-opening-statement-at-ways-and-means-ipab-hearing&catid=89:press -releases-2012&Itemid=500235, accessed June 17, 2012.

30 "One of its architects . . ." Peter Orszag, "Myths about Paul Ryan's Budget," *Washington Post*, August 26, 2012.

31 "In his fiscal year 2013 budget . . ." Marilyn Werber Serafini, "New Ryan Budget Would Transform Medicare and Medicaid," *Kaiser Health News*, March 20, 2012, http://www.kaiserhealthnews.org/Stories/2012/March/20/ryan -budget-medicare-medicaid-republicans.aspx, accessed August 10, 2012.

31 "That same year . . ." Committee for a Responsible Federal Budget, "It Turns Out Ryan and Obama Agree on Putting Medicare in a Budget," March 23, 2012, http://crfb.org/blogs/it-turns-out-ryan-and-obama-agree-putting -medicare-budget, accessed October 31, 2012.

31 "During the 2012 presidential campaign . . ." "The Agenda Project: Granny Off the Cliff," *YouTube*, http://www.youtube.com/watch?v=OGnE83A1Z4U, accessed August 5, 2012.

32 "Goldman Sachs calculated . . ." Carol Gentry, "How Much Are You Worth to HMOs?," *Health News Florida*, October 28, 2011, http://www.healthnews florida.org/top_story/read/how_much_are_you_worth_to_an_hmo, accessed June 29, 2012.

32 "It is used by people . . ." Michael O. Leavitt, "Will Congress Continue a Medicare Scam?" *Wall Street Journal*, July 8, 2008, http://online.wsj.com/ article/SB121556116413437535.html, accessed July 12, 2012.

33 "Almost five years after Congress . . ." Testimony of Omar Perez, "Waste, Fraud and Abuse," U.S. House of Representatives Committee on Energy and Commerce, Subcommittee on Oversight and Investigations, March 2, 2011, http://oig.hhs.gov/testimony/docs/2011/perez_testimony_03022011. pdf, accessed July 20, 2012.

CHAPTER 4

37 "It's getting economies of scale . . ." Geoff Colvin, "Health Care's New Maverick," *Fortune*, August 13, 2012, 98 and 101.

38 "They reported being emotionally . . ." Tait D. Shanafelt et al., "Burnout and Satisfaction with Work-Life Balance among U.S. Physicians Relative to the General U.S. Population," *Archives of Internal Medicine* 172, no. 18 (2012):

1–9, http://archinte.jamanetwork.com/article.aspx?articleid=1351351, accessed August 22, 2012.

39 "They called family doctors' offices . . ." Steve Daniels, "Doctors Who Take Medicare Scarce," *ABC11 Investigates*, May 10, 2012, http://abclocal.go.com/wtvd/story?section=news/abc11_investigates&id=8656615, accessed August 13, 2012.

CHAPTER 5

43 "If the entire development . . ." Trulia, listing for Medicare Drive, Somerset, Kentucky, 42501, MLS 11275, http://www.trulia.com/property/3023982767 --Medicare-Dr-Somerset-KY-42501, accessed January 14, 2012.

44 "The bill that I received . . ." G. D., letter to the editor, *Commonwealth Journal*, June 1, 2011, http://somerset-kentucky.com/letters/x1886881592/Controlling-Medical-Costs, accessed July 17, 2012.

45 "This gives us negotiating . . ." Jeff Sherman, 30th Annual JP Morgan Health Care Conference, January 10, 2012, http://jpmorgan.metameetings .com/webcasts/healthcare12/directlink.php?ticker=LPNT, accessed June 16, 2012.

45 "Additionally, because non-urban . . ." LifePoint, SEC 10-K filing, 2005, 6, http://phx.corporate-ir.net/phoenix.zhtml?c=88004&p=irol-SECText& TEXT=aHR0cDovL2lyLmludC53ZXN0bGF3aW5lc3MuY29tL2Rv Y3VtZW50L3YxLzAwMDA5NTAxNDQtMDctMDctMDAwODg1L3htbA%3d %3d, accessed November 23, 2012.

45 "In June 2011 . . ." The Joint Commission, "Quality Report: Lake Cumberland Regional Hospital," June 28, 2011, http://www.qualitycheck.org/QualityReportHistory.aspx?hcoid=4852, accessed January 15, 2012.

47 "Four months later . . ." Ibid.

48 "When Dr. Renee Hsia . . ." Renee Y. Hsia et al., "Health Care as a 'Market Good'? Appendicitis as a Case Study," *Archives of Internal Medicine* 172, no. 10 (2011): 818–19, http://archinte.jamanetwork.com/article .aspx?articleid=1151669, accessed July 20, 2012.

48 "If a person has the . . ." U.S. Census Bureau, "Quick Facts," http://quick facts.census.gov/qfd/states/06000.html, accessed August 11, 2012.

49 "The cost of a basic . . ." FAIR Health, "FH Medical Cost Lookup," CPT Code 45378, http://fairhealthconsumer.org/medicalcostlookup/cost.aspx, accessed November 22, 2012.

49 "When we pay directly . . ." Paul Ryan, "Consumer Choice Can Save U.S. Health Care," *Bloomberg View*, May 26, 2011, http://www.bloomberg .com/apps/news?pid=2065100&sid=ayyTSE7N87DA, accessed November 22, 2012.

50 "It is about . . ." U.S. Census Bureau, "Quick Facts," http://quickfacts .census.gov/cgi-bin/qfd/extract?2171688, accessed April 2, 2012.

CHAPTER 6

51 "In December 1992 . . ." Frances Leslie Lucas et al., "New Cardiac Surgery Programs Established from 1993 to 2004 Led to Little Increased Access, Substantial Duplication of Services," *Health Affairs*, June 2011, http://content .healthaffairs.org/content/early/2011/06/21/hlthaff.2010.0210.abstract, accessed July 5, 2012.

52 "Duplicative facilities had . . ." Ibid.

52 "Instead, the additional . . ." Thomas W. Concannon et al., "A Percutaneous Coronary Intervention Lab in Every Hospital?," *Circulation*, December 6, 2011, http://circoutcomes.ahajournals.org/content/5/1/14.full, accessed July 5, 2012.

53 "Critics of Medicare . . ." Walter Williams, "Moral Hazards," March 22, 1999, http://econfaculty.gmu.edu/wew/articles/99/Moral-Hazards.htm, accessed July 5, 2012.

53 "Negligence and profusion . . ." Adam Smith, *An Inquiry into the Nature and Causes of the Wealth of Nations* (1776; repr. Edinburgh: Thomas Nelson and Peter Brown, 1827), 311.

53 "In August 2012 . . ." Reed Abelson and Julie Creswell, "Hospital Chain Inquiry Cited Unnecessary Cardiac Work," *New York Times*, August 6, 2012, http://www.nytimes.com/2012/08/07/business/hospital-chain-internal -reports-found-dubious-cardiac-work.html?pagewanted=all, accessed August 10, 2012.

54 "Doctors have implanted . . ." Sana Al-Khatib et al., "Non-Evidence-Based ICD Implantations in the United States," *Journal of the American Medical Association*, 305, no. 1 (2011): 43–49.

55 "The probe was targeted . . ." Centers for Medicare and Medicaid Services, "CMS Announces New Demonstrations to Help Curb Improper Medicare and Medicaid Payments," press release, November 15, 2011, http://www .cms.gov/apps/media/press/factsheet.asp?Counter=4176&intNumPerPage= 10&checkDate=&checkKey=&srchType=1&numDays=3500&srchOpt=0& srchData=&keywordType=All&chkNewsType=6&intPage=&showAll=&p Year=&year=&desc=&cboOrder=date, accessed May 15, 2012.

56 "This estimate apparently . . ." American College of Cardiology, Florida Chapter, "CMS Audit Info: Background Information," http://www.accfl .org/take-action/take-action.html, accessed May 20, 2012. See also American College of Cardiology, Oregon Chapter, *Oregon ACC Newsletter*, November 2011, http://archive.constantcontact.com/fs093/1102399426198/archive/1108869519454.html, accessed November 22, 2012.

56 "*Bloomberg News* reported . . ." Larry Husten, "CMS Tightening the Screws on Unnecessary Procedures in Florida and 10 Other States," *Forbes.com*, December 4, 2011, http://www.forbes.com/sites/larryhusten/2011/12/04/cms-tightening-the-screws-on-unnecessary-procedures-in-florida-and-10-other-states/, accessed September 12, 2012.

56 "Bowing to the pressure . . ." "CMS Demonstration Projects—November 2011," *RAC Force*, January 26, 2012, http://racforce.com/cms-demonstration-news/cms-demonstration-projects/, accessed August 30, 2012.

57 "In a broadside against . . ." Joint Letter to Marilyn B. Tavenner, "RE: CMS' Improper Payments Initiatives," April 3, 2012, http://www.mgma.com/WorkArea/DownloadAsset.aspx?id=1370521&ecid=8589&kc=wac, accessed May 1, 2012.

57 "Seven months later . . ." American Hospital Association, "Hospitals Sue Federal Government for Unfair Medicare Practices," press release, November 1, 2012.

60 "One-third of them . . ." Sabrina K. H. How et al., "Public View on U.S. Health System Organization: A Call for New Directions," *Data Brief*, August 2008, 4, http://www.commonwealth-fund.org/usr_doc/Public_Views_SurveyPg_8-4-08.pdf?section=4056, accessed November 21, 2012.

61 "And why not? . . ." Practice Builders, www.practicebuilders.com, accessed July 3, 2012.

62 "Marketers urge oncologists . . ." Knowledge Driven, "Expanding Oncology's Market Reach," November 8, 2010, http://www.knowledgedriven.com/webisode-provider-series-greater-market-outreach-for-oncology, accessed June 16, 2012.

63 "These numbers don't include . . ." Richard Johnson and Corina Mommaerts, "Will Health Care Costs Bankrupt Aging Boomers?," Urban Institute, February 2010, http://www.urban.org/uploadedpdf/412026_health_care_costs.pdf, accessed May 18, 2012.

64 "In 1981 only . . ." David Himmelstein et al., "Medical Bankruptcy in the United States, 2007: Results of a National Study," *American Journal of Medicine* 20, no. 10 (2009), http://www.washingtonpost.com/wp-srv/politics/documents/american_journal_of_medicine_09.pdf, accessed May 14, 2012.

CHAPTER 7

66 "In 2012 . . ." "Avastin Has Similar Effect to Lucentis in Treating Most Common Cause of Blindness in the Developed World," *Science Daily*, May 6,

2012, http://www.sciencedaily.com/releases/2012/05/120506160147.htm, accessed June 16, 2012.

67 "Seniors paid nearly . . ." Office of the Inspector General, U.S. Department of Health and Human Services, "Medicare Payments for Drugs Used to Treat Wet Age-Related Macular Degeneration," April 2012, http://oig.hhs.gov/oei/reports/oei-03-10-00360.pdf, accessed June 17, 2012.

67 "The federal district court . . ." *Hays v. Leavitt*, U.S. District Court of the District of Columbia, October 16, 2008, https://ecf.dcd.uscourts.gov/cgi-bin/show_public_doc?2008cv1032-22, accessed June 17, 2012.

68 "The nonpartisan Medicare . . ." Letter from Glenn Hackbarth to Vice President Joseph Biden and Speaker of the House of Representatives John Boehner, "Report to the Congress: Medicare Payment Policy," March 15, 2012, http://www.medpac.gov/documents/Mar12_EntireReport.pdf, accessed December 1, 2012.

68 "Twelve million Medicare . . ." Medicare Payment Advisory Commission, "Report to the Congress: Medicare Payment Policy," March 2012, http://www.medpac.gov/documents/Mar12_EntireReport.pdf, accessed June 18, 2012.

68 "According to the Medicare . . ." Ibid., 330.

69 "The health insurance . . ." Letter from Lynn Gibson to Kathleen Sebelius, "RE: Medicare Advantage Quality Bonus Payment Demonstration," July 11, 2012, http://www.gao.gov/assets/600/592303.pdf, accessed July 14, 2012.

71 "It has a backlog . . ." Whet Moser, "Illinois's Medicaid Mess," *Chicago Magazine*, February 20, 2012, http://www.chicagomag.com/Chicago-Magazine/The-312/February-2012/Illinois-Medicaid-Mess/, accessed June 21, 2012.

71 "If nothing changes . . ." Christopher Wills, "Senate Gets Medicaid Lessons," *Northwest Herald*, March 23, 2012, http://www.nwherald.com/2012/03/22/sens-get-medicaid-lesson/axqyxxd/?page=1, accessed June 21, 2012.

71 "A medical equipment . . ." Joshua Chaffin, "Greek Business Looks for Life in 'Dead Economy,'" *Financial Times*, June 20, 2012, 4.

CHAPTER 8

76 "Hospice Care of Kansas . . ." *United States of America, ex rel., and Beverly Landis v. Hospice Care of Kansas and Voyager HospiceCare*, Case No. 06-2455-CM, http://docs.justia.com/cases/federal/district-courts/kansas/ksdce/2:2006cv02455/58796/68/0.pdf?1291802425, accessed July 25, 2012.

77 "According to court documents . . ." Ibid.

78 "It made a lot of money . . ." Peter Waldman, "Aunt Midge Not Dying in Hospice Reveals $14 Billion Market," *Bloomberg*, December 5, 2011,

http://www.bloomberg.com/news/2011-12-06/hospice-care-revealed-as
-14-billion-u-s-market.html, accessed September 14, 2012.

78 "The president of . . ." Harden Health Care, "Meet Our Executive Team," http://www.hardenhealthcare.com/executive-team.php, accessed July 12, 2012.

78 "The same year . . ." Waldman, "Aunt Midge Not Dying in Hospice."

81 "Large hospices owned . . ." Michael J. McCue and Jon M. Thompson, "Operational and Financial Performance of Publicly Traded Hospice Companies," *Journal of Palliative Medicine* 8, no. 6 (December 2005): 1196, http://online.liebertpub.com/doi/abs/10.1089/jpm.2005.8.1196, accessed July 11, 2012.

81 "It doesn't matter . . ." Melissa Carlson et al., "Hospice Care Operated by For-Profit Companies Provide a Narrower Range of Services," *Medical Care* 42, no. 5 (May 2004): 432–38, http://news.yale.edu/2004/04/20/hospice -care-operated-profit-companies-provides-narrower-range-services, accessed July 10, 2012.

82 "In January 2012 . . ." U.S. Department of Justice, "U.S. Files Complaint against National Chain of Hospice Providers Alleging False Claims on the Medicare Program," press release, January 3, 2012, http://www.justice.gov/ opa/pr/2012/January/12-civ-001.html, accessed July 30, 2012.

83 "In 2009 a Birmingham . . ." U.S. Department of Justice, "Alabama-Based Hospice Company Pays U.S. $24.7 Million to Settle Health Care Fraud Claims," press release, January 15, 2009, http://www.justice.gov/opa/ pr/2009/January/09-civ-043.html, accessed July 28, 2012.

83 "In 2006 national . . ." U.S. Department of Justice, "Odyssey Healthcare to Pay U.S. $12.9 Million to Resolve Hospice Fraud Case," press release, July 13, 2006, http://www.justice.gov/opa/pr/2006/July/06_civ_430.html, accessed July 30, 2012.

83 "Wald and her . . ." Florence Wald, interviewed by Monica Mills, Connecticut Women's Hall of Fame, June 10, 2003, http://cwhf.org/media/ upload/files/Transcripts/Wald%20Interview%20Transcript.pdf, accessed July 28, 2012.

84 "Usually, the patient . . ." Florence Wald, interviewed by Jane Kolleeny, National Prison Hospice Association, http://npha.org/npha-articles/interviews -news/interview-with-florence-wald/, accessed July 31, 2012.

84 "The Wharton Business . . ." Florence Wald, interviewed by Monica Mills.

85 "If you need nursing . . ." Government Accountability Office, "Nursing Homes: Complexity of Private Investment Purchases Demonstrates Need for CMS to Improve the Usability and Completeness of Ownership Data," October 27, 2010, http://www.gao.gov/htext/d10710.html, accessed November 22, 2012.

86 "Three of them . . ." U.S. Senate, Committee on Finance, "Baucus, Grassley Uncover Gaming of the Medicare System by For-Profit Home Care Companies," press release, October 3, 2011, http://www.finance.senate.gov/newsroom/chairman/release/?id=e32d81a2-da53-4d9c-bccc-1c50a1f33f5e, accessed November 22, 2012.

86 "JPMorgan brokers . . ." Susanne Craig and Jessica Silver-Greenberg, "Former Brokers Say JPMorgan Favored Selling Bank's Own Funds over Others," *New York Times*, July 2, 2012, http://dealbook.nytimes.com/2012/07/02/ex-brokers-say-jpmorgan-favored-selling-banks-own-funds-over-others/, accessed November 22, 2012.

CHAPTER 9

91 "Researchers who studied . . ." P. P. Garg et al., "Effect of the Ownership of Dialysis Facilities on Patients' Survival and Referral for Transplantation," *New England Journal of Medicine* 341, no. 22 (November 25, 1999): 1653–60, http://www.ncbi.nlm.nih.gov/pubmed/10572154, accessed July 10, 2012.

91 "For-profit dialysis . . ." Mae Thamer et al., "Dialysis Facility Ownership and Epoetin Dosing in Patients Receiving Hemodialysis," *Journal of the American Medical Association* 297, no. 15 (April 18, 2007): 1667–74, http://jama.jamanetwork.com/article.aspx?articleid=206629, accessed September 4, 2012.

92 "Its actions harmed . . ." Peter Whoriskey, "Anemia Drugs Made Billions but at What Cost?," *Washington Post*, July 20, 2012, http://www.washingtonpost.com/business/economy/anemia-drug-made-billions-but-at-what-cost/2012/07/19/gJQAX5yqwW_story.html, accessed September 9, 2012.

92 "Medical experts . . ." Ibid.

92 "Amgen stocks jumped . . ." Ibid.

93 "The groundbreaking research . . ." Food and Drug Administration, "Modified Dosing Recommendations to Improve the Safe Use of Erythropoiesis-Stimulating Agents (ESAs) in Chronic Kidney Disease," June 24, 2011, http://www.fda.gov/Drugs/DrugSafety/ucm259639.htm, accessed July 13, 2012. See also A. K. Singh, "Is There a Deleterious Effect of Erythropoietin in End-Stage Renal Disease?," *Kidney International* 80, no. 6 (September 2011): 569–71.

93 "More than a decade . . ." Food and Drug Administration, "Modified Dosing Recommendations."

93 "The following year, DaVita . . ." Michael Booth and Christopher Osher, "Denver-Based DaVita Settles Case on Overuse of Kidney Care Drug," *Denver Post*, July 4, 2012, http://www.denverpost.com/news/ci_21002816/denver-based-davita-settles-case-overuse-kidney-care, accessed September 3, 2012.

93 "More than 20 percent . . ." Tom Parker and Theodore Steinman, "Renal Policy: Changing the Models and Measurements of Dialysis Care," *Nephrology News and Issues*, April 27, 2011, http://www.nephrologynews.com/renal-policy/article/renal-policy-changing-the-models-and-measurements-of-dialysis-care, accessed July 13, 2012.

CHAPTER 10

100 "For his reelection . . ." Kevin Roose, "Wall St.'s Dinner with Obama: Hold the Scorn," *DealB%k*, June 23, 2011, http://dealbook.nytimes.com/2011/06/23/wall-streets-dinner-with-obama-hold-the-scorn/, accessed July 14, 2012.

100 "The federal government spends . . ." Congressional Budget Office, "Monthly Budget Review," October 5, 2012, http://www.cbo.gov/publication/43656, accessed November 22, 2012.

100 "He traveled to Washington . . ." Steven Baker, "Failed Implanted Medical Devices—Senate Hearing Tuesday 11/15/11," Failed Implant Device Alliance, http://fida-advocate.blogspot.com/2011/11/failed-implanted-medical-devices-senate.html, accessed July 12, 2012.

103 "The health care industry . . ." Center for Responsive Politics, "Lobbying: Health Sector Profile," *OpenSecrets.org*, http://www.opensecrets.org/lobby/indus.php?id=H&year=2012, accessed July 4, 2012.

104 "Drug companies and hospitals . . ." Ibid.

104 "The cuts would threaten . . ." American Hospital Association, "Ads Urge Congress to Reject Cuts That Hurt Patient Care and Hospital Jobs," *AHA News*, November 1, 2011, http://www.ahanews.com/ahanews_app/jsp/display.jsp?dcrpath=AHANEWS/AHANewsNowArticle/data/ann_110111_ads&domain=AHANEWS, accessed November 3, 2012.

104 "The American Hospital Association . . ." Tracy Jan, "Hospitals Push Age Hike for Medicare," *Boston Globe*, September 30, 2011, http://www.bostonglobe.com/news/nation/2011/09/29/hospital-executives-lobby-raise-medicare-eligibility-age/Y9a91Pm90pqMMjRukRF8AJ/story.html, accessed September 5, 2012.

104 "Bernie Sanders . . ." Bernie Sanders, "The Hospital Lobby vs. Medicare," press release, October 5, 2011, http://sanders.senate.gov/newsroom/news/?id=C49C1A83-0F45-4B62-B1D3-5D1985BE770B, accessed August 25, 2012.

105 "With inadequate premarket . . ." Gregory Curfman, Testimony before the Subcommittee on Oversight and Investigations, Committee on Energy and Commerce, House of Representatives, July 20, 2011, 73, http://www

.gpo.gov/fdsys/pkg/CHRG-112hhrg73314/html/CHRG-112hhrg73314.htm, accessed November 22, 2012.

106 "She told a congressional . . ." Katherine Korgaokar, Testimony before the Senate Committee on Aging, April 13, 2011, http://aging.senate.gov/events/hr233kk.pdf, accessed December 27, 2011.

107 "Sixty-eight percent . . ." Consumer Reports, "Consumer Reports Poll: Americans Overwhelmingly Support Strong Medical Device Safety Oversight," press release, March 20, 2012, http://www.consumersunion.org/pub/core_health_care/018376.html, accessed November 23, 2012.

107 "Dr. Curfman of the . . ." Curfman, testimony before the Subcommittee on Oversight and Investigations, 4.

107 "Not a single new . . ." Barry Meier and Janet Roberts, "Venture Capitalists Put Money on Easing Medical Device Rules," *New York Times*, October 25, 2011, http://www.nytimes.com/2011/10/26/business/venture-capitalists-join-push-to-ease-fda-rules-for-medical-device-industry.html, accessed August 1, 2012.

108 "Mr. Paulsen's campaign . . ." Ibid.

108 "Democrats on the congressional . . ." Letter from Henry Waxman et al. to Frank Upton et al., October 12, 2011, http://democrats.energycommerce.house.gov/index.php?q=news/energy-and-commerce-democratic-leadership-calls-for-further-examination-of-fda-medical-device-r, accessed December 26, 2011.

108 "A study funded by National Institutes of . . ." National Institutes of Health, "NIH Stroke Prevention Trial Has Immediate Implications for Clinical Practice," news release, September 7, 2011, http://www.nih.gov/news/health/sep2011/ninds-07.htm, accessed November 22, 2012.

109 "Congressman Adam Kinzinger . . ." Eric Paulsen, "Paulsen, Altmire Lead Bipartisan Effort to Increase Efficiency at the FDA," press release, October 14, 2011, http://paulsen.house.gov/press-releases/paulsen-altmire-lead-bipartisan-effort-to-increase-efficiency-at-the-fda/, accessed September 12, 2012.

109 "The cost today of engineering . . ." Arundhati Parmar, "Omar Ishrak's Medtronic: Bigger in India, with More R&D Hiring in Asia," *Medcity News*, September 11, 2011, http://www.medcitynews.com/2011/09/omar-ishraks-medtronic-more-prominent-in-india-rd-hiring-in-asia/, accessed August 15, 2012.

109 "Six months earlier, Medtronic . . ." "Medtronic Inaugurates Its New Regional Headquarters Building in Greater China," press release, March 9, 2011, http://wwwp.medtronic.com/Newsroom/NewsReleaseDetails.do?itemId=1299604172619&lang=en_U.S., accessed August 12, 2012.

110 "The medical device industry . . ." Brett Norman, "FDA Bill No Model for Bipartisanship," *Politico,* June 25, 2012, http://www.politico.com/news/stories/0612/77815.html, accessed July 14, 2012.

CHAPTER 11

120 "About 79,200 Medicare . . ." U.S. Department of Health and Human Services, Office of the Inspector General, "Adverse Events in Hospitals, National Incidence among Medicare Beneficiaries," November 2010, http://oig.hhs.gov/oei/reports/oei-06-09-00090.pdf, accessed June 6, 2012.

123 "Medicare posts the hospital . . ." See U.S. Department of Health and Human Services, "Healthcare-Associated Infections," http://www.hospital compare.hhs.gov/Data/RCD/Healthcare-Associated-Infections.aspx, accessed September 4, 2012.

124 "Up to 12 percent . . ." Richard Hawkins et al., "A Multi-method Study of Needs for Physician Assessment: Implications for Education and Regulation," *Journal of Continuing Education in the Health Professions* 29, no. 4 (2009): 220–34.

124 "Once I'm finished . . ." Hawkins et al., "A Multi-method Study," 228.

125 "A professional license . . ." *O'Brien v. O'Brien,* Court of Appeals of New York State, 1985, http://www.courts.state.ny.us/reporter/archives/o_brien .htm, accessed September 12, 2012.

125 "A trenchant and revealing . . ." Donald Trunkey and Richard Botney, "Assessing Competency: A Tale of Two Professions," *Journal of the American College of Surgeons* 192, no. 3 (March 2001): 385–95, http://www.journalacs .org/article/S1072-7515(01)00770-0/abstract, accessed August 16, 2012.

126 "Yet state medical boards . . ." Alan Levine, Robert Oshel, and Sidney Wolfe, "State Medical Boards Fail to Discipline Doctors with Hospital Actions against Them," Public Citizen, March 2011, http://www.citizen.org/documents/1937.pdf, accessed July 13, 2012.

126 "The public can access . . ." Office of the Inspector General, "Exclusions Program," http://oig.hhs.gov/exclusions/index.asp, accessed July 15, 2012.

127 "The stay has been lifted . . ." Levine, Oshel, and Wolfe, "State Medical Boards Fail to Discipline Doctors," 4.

128 "A handful of GPOs . . ." Patricia Earl and Philip Zweig, "Connecting the Dots: How Anticompetitive Contracting Practices, Kickbacks, and Self-Dealing by Hospital Group Purchasing Organizations (GPOs) Caused the U.S. Drug Shortage," *Care and Cost,* February 14, 2012, http://careandcost .com/2012/02/14/connecting-the-dots-how-anticompetitive-contracting -practices-kickbacks-and-self-dealing-by-hospital-group-purchasing-organi zations-gpos-caused-the-u-s-drug-shortage/, accessed June 9, 2012.

128 "A jury awarded more . . ." *Kinetic Concepts, Inc. v. Hillenbrand Indus., Inc.*, 95-CV-0755 (W.D. Tex., August 31, 2000), as cited in Robert E. Bloch, Scott P. Perlman, and Jay S. Brown, "An Analysis of Group Purchasing Organizations' Contracting Practices under the Antitrust Laws: Myth and Reality," http://www.ftc.gov/ogc/healthcarehearings/docs/030926bloch .pdf, accessed June 7, 2012.

128 "A trenchant analysis . . ." Earl and Zweig, "Connecting the Dots."

129 "Medicare made forty-eight billion . . ." Kay Daly and Kathleen King, "Improper Payments: Reported Medicare Improper Payments and Key Remediation Steps," Government Accountability Office, July 28, 2011, p. 1, http:// www.gao.gov/new.items/d11842t.pdf, accessed August 16, 2012.

130 "In an interview on . . ." "Americans Concerned about Government Corruption: Interview with Frank Newport," *Marketplace*, August 2, 2012, http://www.marketplace.org/topics/elections/attitude-check/americans -concerned-about-government-corruption, accessed August 16, 2012.

132 "In fall 2011 . . ." Alan Bavley, "Bad Medicine: Doctors with Many Malpractice Payments Keep Clean Licenses," *Kansas City Star*, September 4, 2011, http://www.kansascity.com/2011/09/04/3362970/bad-medicine .html, accessed July 16, 2012.

132 "Instead of conducting . . ." Letter from Charles Grassley to Kathleen Sebelius, November 3, 2011, http://www.grassley.senate.gov/about/ upload/2011_11_03-CEG-to-HHS-NPDB.pdf, accessed July 14, 2012.

133 "'As a result of these stories' . . ." Letter from Charles Ornstein et al. to Mary Wakefield, September 15, 2011, https://www.nasw.org/sites/default/ files/Letter%20attachments.pdf, accessed July 16, 2012.

133 "For most of these years . . ." Alan Bavley, "Secrecy Protects Doctors with Long Histories of Problems," *Kansas City Star,* December 17, 2011, http:// www.kansascity.com/2011/12/17/3325411/secrecy-protects-problem -doctors.html, accessed July 14, 2012.

CHAPTER 12

135 "The Project on Government . . ." Adam Zagorin, "Wall Street in Washington: Insider Access," Project on Government Oversight, December 8, 2011, http://www.pogo.org/pogo-files/alerts/government-corruption/wall -street-in-washington-gc-ii-20111208.html, accessed August 8, 2012.

136 "They got to probe . . ." Ibid.

139 "According to the *Wall Street Journal* . . ." Brody Mullins and Susan Pulliam, "Inside Capitol, Investor Access Yields Rich Tips," *Wall Street Journal,*

December 20, 2011, A1 and A16, http://online.wsj.com/article/SB100014 24052970204844504577100260349084878.html, accessed August 31, 2012.

139 "I think it's such . . ." David Morgan, "Lieberman: Public Option Is 'Wrong,'" *CBS Face the Nation*, November 3, 2009, http://www.cbsnews .com/2100-3460_162-5484246.html, accessed August 5,2012.

139 "According to the company's website . . ." JNK Securities, "U.S. Government Policy," http://www.jnksecurities.com/services/us-government -policy, accessed August 3, 2012.

139 "True to its advertisement . . ." Mullins and Pulliam, "Inside Capitol."

139 "Almost two and a half years . . ." Daniel Wagner, "Supreme Court Decision Causes Hospital Stocks to Jump," *Huffington Post*, June 28, 2012, http://www.huffingtonpost.com/2012/06/28/supreme-court-health-care -decision-stocks-jump_n_1634067.html, accessed August 9, 2012.

142 "Never has the need . . ." Letter from Jamie Court and Carmen Balber to Bill Frist, "RE: Medical Malpractice Proposal's Benefits to Your Family's Hospitals Mandate Your Recusal," February 20, 2004, Consumer Watchdog, http://www.consumerwatchdog.org/node/8776, accessed August 6, 2012.

143 "In 2012 Bill Frist's brother . . ." "Thomas Frist, Jr. and Family," *Forbes*, September 2012, http://www.forbes.com/profile/thomas-frist/, accessed July 31, 2012.

CHAPTER 13

145 "Obama garnered . . ." Center for Responsive Politics, "Health Sector Totals to Candidates," http://www.opensecrets.org/pres12/sectors.php?sector=H, accessed December 5, 2012.

145 "Romney vowed to repeal . . ." Ibid.

145 "More than forty-seven . . ." Paul Blumenthal and Sam Stein, "Mitt Romney Builds Fundraising List on Health Care Ruling, Obama Campaign Says It Raised More," *Huffington Post*, http://www.huffingtonpost.com/2012/06/29/ mitt-romney-fundraising-health-care-barack-obama_n_1637677.html, accessed September 5, 2012.

146 "If you are a fiscal conservative . . ." Newt Gingrich, "Conservatives Should Vote 'Yes' on Medicare," *Wall Street Journal*, November 20, 2003, http://www.aei.org/print/conservatives-should-vote-yes-on-medicare, accessed September 12, 2012.

146 "During the Medicare drug . . ." "Newt Gingrich on Health Care," *PoliGu.com*, January 27, 2012, http://www.thepoliticalguide.com/Profiles/ House/Georgia/Newt_Gingrich/Views/Health_Care/, accessed December 1, 2012.

146 "He gathered about . . ." Julie Bykowicz and Kristin Jensen, "Gingrich 'Loophole' Offers Lobbyist Access for Consultant Cash," *Bloomberg*, December 29, 2011, http://www.bloomberg.com/news/2011-12-29/gingrich-loophole-offers-lobbyist-access-for-consultant-cash.html, accessed August 3, 2012.

146 "Fast-forward ten . . ." "2011 Annual Report of the Boards of Trustees of the Federal Hospital Insurance and Federal Supplementary Medical Insurance Trust Funds," May 13, 2011, 146, http://www.cms.gov/Research-Statistics-Data-and-Systems/Statistics-Trends-and-Reports/ReportsTrustFunds/downloads/tr2011.pdf, accessed August 16, 2012.

147 "Top-brass . . ." "Gingrich Think Tank Collected Millions from Health-Care Industry," *Washington Post*, http://www.washingtonpost.com/politics/gingrich-think-tank-collected-millions-from-health-care-industry/2011/11/16/gIQAcd72VN_story_1.html, accessed August 16, 2012.

147 "You have Medicare . . ." Igor Volsky and Scott Keyes, "Rick Santorum: Medicare Is 'Crushing' the 'Entire Health Care System in This Country,'" *Think Progress*, January 3, 2012, http://thinkprogress.org/health/2012/01/03/396407/rick-santorum-medicare-is-crushing-the-entire-health-care-system-in-this-country/, accessed January 14, 2012.

147 "One of the solutions . . ." *Meet the Press* Transcript for Jan. 8, 2012, *MSNBC.com*, January 8, 2012, http://www.msnbc.msn.com/id/45917518/ns/meet_the_press-transcripts/t/meet-press-transcript-jan/, accessed September 9, 2012.

147 "Santorum received . . ." Mike McIntire and Michael Luo, "After Santorum Left Senate, Familiar Hands Reached Out," *New York Times*, January 5, 2012, http://www.nytimes.com/2012/01/06/us/politics/after-senate-santorums-beneficiaries-became-benefactors.html?_r=1, accessed July 17, 2012.

147 "Employees at health . . ." Center for Responsive Politics, "Presidential Candidate Comparison: Top Contributors, 2012 Cycle," *OpenSecrets.org*, http://www.opensecrets.org/pres12/contriball.php?cycle=2012, accessed July 17, 2102.

147 "While Santorum was critical . . ." Center for Responsive Politics, "Donor Lookup Results; Donor Occupation: Universal Health Services," http://www.opensecrets.org/pres12/search.php?cid=&name=&employ=universal+health+services&state=%28all%29&zip=%28any+zip%29&submit=OK&amt=a&sort=A, accessed September 1, 2012.

148 "He acknowledged his soft . . ." "Ron Paul: 'Freedom Is a Young Idea and We're Throwing It Away,'" *PBS NewsHour,* July 20, 2011, http://www.pbs.org/newshour/bb/politics/july-dec11/ronpaul_07-20.html, accessed July 17, 2012.

148 "Huntsman agreed . . ." "Romney, Santorum, Others Call for Medicare 'Premium Support' in New Hampshire GOP Debate," January 9, 2012,

Kaiser Health News, http://www.kaiserhealthnews.org/Multimedia/2012/ January/GOP-debate-meet-the-press.aspx, accessed July 31, 2012.

148 "One of the top contributors . . ." "Top Presidential Contributors," Reuters, http://graphics.thomsonreuters.com/11/11/US_CANDIDATE CONTRIB1111_VT.html, accessed August 1, 2012.

148 "It has its sights . . ." "Fresenius Medical Care in China," Fresenius, http://www.fresenius.com/749.htm, accessed September 1, 2012.

149 "Total contributions . . ." Center for Responsive Politics, "Presidential Candidates: Health Sector Totals."

149 "Roemer told supporters . . ." "Buddy Roemer: GOP Pres. Candidate Who Backs Occupy, Campaign Finance Reform, Excluded from Debates," *Democracy Now!,* January 6, 2012, http://www.democracynow.org/2012/1/6/ buddy_roemer_gop_pres_candidate_who, accessed July 19, 2012.

CHAPTER 14

153 "That's why Americans . . ." Donald Trump, *Time to Get Tough: Making America #1 Again* (Washington, DC: Regnery, 2011), 121.

153 "Stanford University economist . . ." John B. Taylor, *First Principles: Five Keys to Restoring America's Prosperity* (New York: W. W. Norton, 2012), 177.

154 "A different user . . ." Managed Senior Services, "Testamonials," http://managedseniorservices.com/testimonials.htm, accessed December 31, 2011.

154 "Most boomers and seniors . . ." National Council on Aging and UnitedHealthcare, "Survey of Boomers and Seniors," August 2011, http://www .ncoa.org/assets/files/pdf/9-16-11-UHC-NCOA-Survey-Results-Report -FINAL.pdf, accessed July 20, 2012.

154 "Faced with an . . ." Harvard Medical School, "Complex Choices in Medicare Advantage Program May Overwhelm Seniors, Study Finds," press release, August 18, 2011, http://www.eurekalert.org/pub_releases/2011-08/ hms-cci081611.php, accessed June 17, 2012. See also J. Michael McWilliams et al., "Complex Medicare Advantage Choices May Overwhelm Seniors— Especially Those with Impaired Decision Making," *Health Affairs* 30, no. 9 (September 2011): 1786–94.

155 "Also consider that . . ." Alzheimer's Association, "2012 Alzheimer's Disease Facts and Figures," http://www.alz.org/downloads/facts_figures_2012 .pdf, accessed June 17, 2012. See also Mayur Desai et al., "Trends in Vision and Hearing among Older Americans," Centers for Disease Control and Prevention, National Center for Health Statistics, March 2001, http://www .cdc.gov/nchs/data/ahcd/agingtrends/02vision.pdf, accessed June 18, 2012.

155 "The center helped . . ." Medicare Rights Center, "Why Consumers Disenroll from Medicare Private Plans," Summer 2010, http://www.medi carerights.org/pdf/Why-Consumers-Disenroll-from-MA.pdf, accessed July 20, 2012.

156 "This is why the Nobel . . ." Kenneth J. Arrow, "Uncertainty and the Welfare Economics of Medical Care," *American Economic Review* 53, no 5. (December 1963): 941–73, http://www.who.int/bulletin/volumes/82/2/ PHCBP.pdf, accessed July 20, 2012.

156 "No issue is more critical . . ." Rick Perry, *Fed Up!: Our Fight to Save America from Washington* (New York: Little, Brown, 2010), 78.

157 "That's just not right . . ." "Prescriptions and Profits," *60 Minutes*, December 5, 2007, http://www.cbsnews.com/8301-18560_162-605700.html, accessed December 1, 2012.

158 "A Canadian pharmacist . . ." Rebecca Leung, "Prescriptions and Profit," *60 Minutes*, December 5, 2007, http://www.cbsnews.com/2100-18560_162 -605700.html, accessed September 3, 2012.

159 "They thought Roosevelt . . ." Franz H. Messerli, "This Day 50 Years Ago," *New England Journal of Medicine* 332, no. 15 (April 13, 1995): 1038–39.

160 "Leading doctors say . . ." National Priorities Partnership, *National Priorities and Goals*, 2008, http://www.pcpcc.net/files/NPP_Report_111809.pdf, accessed December 1, 2012.

160 "The night before his surgery . . ." David S. Jones, "Visions of a Cure: Visualization, Clinical Trials, and Controversies in Cardiac Therapeutics, 1968–1998," *Isis* 91, no. 3 (2000): 504–41.

161 "People with moderate . . ." Dean Ornish et al., "Intensive Lifestyle Changes for Reversal of Coronary Heart Disease," *Journal of the American Medical Association* 280, no. 23 (December 16, 1998): 2001–7, http://jama .jamanetwork.com/article.aspx?articleid=188274, accessed June 26, 2012.

161 "The plan is to help . . ." Alona Pulde and Matthew Lederman, "Practice Spotlight: Whole Foods Market Wellness Clubs," *Lifestyle Medicine in Action*, December 2011, http://www.lifestylemedicine.org/wholefoodsmarket, accessed July 31, 2012.

CHAPTER 15

165 "The average time . . ." John Melloy, "Is the Buy and Hold Strategy Officially Dead?," *CNBC.com*, June 25, 2012, http://www.cnbc.com/ id/47947707/Is_the_Buy_Hold_Stock_Strategy_Officially_Dead. See also Alan M. Newman, "HFT Wins, Investors Lose: The Greatest Stock Market

Mania of All Time," *Crosscurrents*, October 10, 2012, http://www.cross-currents.net/charts.htm, accessed June 30, 2012.

165 "The citizenry has lost . . ." "NYSE CEO: Investors Have Lost Confidence in the Exchanges," Fox Business, video, June 20, 2012, http://video .foxbusiness.com/v/1698940747001/nyse-ceo-investors-have-lost-confidence -in-exchanges/, accessed June 26, 2012.

166 "Restoring that faith critically requires . . ." Aspen Institute, "Overcoming Short-termism: A Call for a More Responsible Approach to Investment and Business Management," September 9, 2009, http://www.aspeninstitute .org/sites/default/files/content/images/Overcoming%20Short-termism%20 AspenCVSG%2015dec09.pdf, accessed June 26, 2012.

168 "What I want to do is . . ." Harry Truman, "Remarks at the National Health Assembly Dinner," May 1, 1948, http://www.trumanlibrary.org/ publicpapers/viewpapers.php?pid=1612, accessed June 26, 2012.

169 "The financial gurus say . . ." Aspen Institute, "Overcoming Short-termism," 2.

170 "The stock-market gurus say . . ." Ibid.

171 "The stock-market gurus say . . ." Ibid.

172 "The driving dream of our adviser/agents . . ." John C. Bogle, "The Fiduciary Principle: No Man Can Serve Two Masters," Presentation to Columbia University School of Business, April 1, 2009, http://www.vanguard.com/ bogle_site/sp20090401.html, accessed December 1, 2012.

172 "Spending enormous amounts on advertising . . ." Ibid.

174 "The loss and suffering inflicted . . ." Justice Harlan Fiske Stone, address to the University of Michigan Law School, 1934, *Harvard Law Review,* 1934.

176 "The law governing corporations . . ." Robert Hinckley, "How Corporate Law Inhibits Social Responsibility," *Business Ethics*, January/February 2002, http://www.medialens.org/articles/the_articles/articles_2002/rh_corporate_ responsibility.html, accessed July 22, 2012.

176 "Similarly, everyone who works . . ." Ibid.

CHAPTER 16

179 "The editors opined . . ." "Health Care Entitlements," *New York Times*, November 28, 2012, http://www.nytimes.com/2012/11/29/opinion/ health-care-entitlements.html, accessed December 1, 2012.

180 "This will save $15 billion . . ." Congressional Budget Office, "Raising the Ages of Eligibility for Medicare and Social Security," January 2012, 6, http://www.cbo.gov/sites/default/files/cbofiles/attachments/01-10-2012 -Medicare_SS_EligibilityAgesBrief.pdf, accessed December 1, 2012.

Index

About the Authors

Rosemary Gibson is a leading authority on U.S. health care. At the Robert Wood Johnson Foundation, she designed and led national initiatives to improve health care quality and safety. She was vice president of the Economic and Social Research Institute and served as senior associate at the American Enterprise Institute. She is principal author of *The Battle Over Health Care*, *Wall of Silence*, and *The Treatment Trap*. She serves as an editor for JAMA Internal Medicine.

Janardan Prasad Singh is an economist at the World Bank. He has been a member of the International Advisory Council for several prime ministers of India. He worked on economic policy at the American Enterprise Institute and on foreign policy at the United Nations. He has also written extensively on health care, social policy, and economic development, and was a member of the Board of Contributors of the *Wall Street Journal*. He is coauthor of *The Battle Over Health Care*, *Wall of Silence*, and *The Treatment Trap*.